All My Patients Are Under the Bed

DR. LOUIS J. CAMUTI

WITH

MARILYN AND HASKEL FRANKEL

A FIRESIDE BOOK

Published by Simon & Schuster Inc.

New York London Toronto Sydney Tokyo Singapore

COPYRIGHT © 1980 BY DR. LOUIS J. CAMUTI,
HASKEL FRANKEL AND MARILYN FRANKEL

FIRST FIRESIDE EDITION, 1985

PUBLISHED BY SIMON & SCHUSTER, INC.
SIMON & SCHUSTER BUILDING
ROCKEFELLER CENTER
1230 AVENUE OF THE AMERICAS
NEW YORK, NEW YORK 10020

FIRESIDE AND COLOPHON ARE REGISTERED TRADEMARKS OF
SIMON & SCHUSTER, INC.

DESIGNED BY EVE METZ

MANUFACTURED IN THE UNITED STATES OF AMERICA

7 9 10 8 6
12   Pbk.

LIBRARY OF CONGRESS CATALOGING IN PUBLICATION DATA

CAMUTI, LOUIS J.
ALL MY PATIENTS ARE UNDER THE BED.
1. CAMUTI, LOUIS J. 2. VETERINARIANS—NEW YORK
(CITY)—BIOGRAPHY. 3. CATS—DISEASES. I. FRANKEL,
MARILYN, JOINT AUTHOR. II. FRANKEL, HASKEL, JOINT
AUTHOR.III. TITLE.
SF613.C35A33   636.8'089'0924 [B]   80-14728

ISBN: 0-671- 24271-7
ISBN: 0-671-55450-6 Pbk.

I am most grateful to Phyllis Levy and Joni Evans for standing guard over this book while I was ruminating. Without their help and direction my work would have been more difficult. I want to thank Marilyn and Hank Frankel for tailing me for so many months without complaint and for telling my story faithfully. And, finally, many thanks to Carl Brandt for needling me into doing it.

—*Louis J. Camuti*

We, his collaborators on the hardcover edition of *All My Patients Are Under the Bed* dedicate this edition to the memory of our dear friend, Louis J. Camuti. A loving but crusty man, Lou died as he had lived, in the service of his patients. On February 2, 1981, with his beloved wife Alexandra by his side, Lou was driving home to Mount Vernon after a day in New York City. He had gone into town for an adjustment on his pacemaker and to see one of his cat patients. Suddenly, he veered off the road. When the car finally stopped, Alex realized that Lou was dead.

As he lives on in the hearts and minds of family, so he lives with us. And probably with all the Nicodemuses and Oswillas who hissed and spat at the loving care he gave them.

—*Marilyn and Haskel Frankel*

This book is dedicated to my wife Alexandra, my daughter Nina, my niece Dorothy, my daughter-in-law Grace and to the memory of my son, Louis J., Jr., who is resting in the glory of heaven.

FOREWORD

by Haskel Frankel

I DON'T KNOW if dog people know other dog people, or if parakeet people know other parakeet people. But cat people always seem to know other cat people. I think we seek each other out, and though we never really say it to each other, we consider ourselves superior to people who don't have or appreciate cats. I think what makes us feel superior is not that we have a cat in our homes, but that a cat has found us acceptable to live with. There's a thrill in that that a dog owner will never know.

Love from a dog seems such an easy thing. Once a dog has given its love, that love is a constant. The dog is ever there, ready with licks and leaps whenever a human being requires them. That may impress dog people. To a cat person it isn't much. It is almost cheap, it's so easily come by.

But love from a cat is special. When a cat is in the mood, it may give a lick or two with its rough tongue or it may leap into a lap and settle down. But none of these small miracles occurs because some human being has snapped his or her fingers or whistled. To a cat, human beings are an inferior, servile race, always to be kept in their places, with occasional rewards if they perform well. To love a cat is uphill work, and therefore very rewarding.

This special but unspoken bond that exists between cat people explains all sorts of strange phenomena that take place in any big city. Like the sudden swooping raids that occur in supermarkets the minute a kitty litter sale begins or when the little cans of cat food that are usually sold for 35 cents go on sale at "3 for

9

$1.00." Did you ever notice how quickly the shelves empty, and yet no telephone calls have been made between cat owners in advance of the sale?

All of this is to explain how my wife Marilyn and I knew Dr. Louis J. Camuti when our cat Balaban took ill, though until that black Monday morning we had never required a veterinarian in New York City. Our boys (Balaban has a brother, Eartha Katz) had their checkups and shots on Saturdays in Connecticut. But one morning, Balaban wouldn't come out from under the bed, a milky substance trickling from one eye.

The only veterinarian in New York City I had ever heard of was Dr. Camuti. I took the telephone book and riffled through to the C's, found his name, telephoned and left my name and number with his answering service.

"I'll have the doctor call," the service said and clicked off.

I spent the morning sitting on the sofa with a cold cup of coffee on the table in front of me, watching Balaban, a black-and-white shadow now hiding under the dining table. Eartha was sound asleep in a patch of sunlight on the living-room rug.

Ask anyone who has ever loved a cat. There is no sound more deep, more all-enveloping than the silence of a sick cat. The emptiness, the hollowness, reaches out and fills the air of a house while the animal sits in the middle, folded into itself, unreachable, unresponding.

I found myself looking at my wristwatch every few minutes. Where was this Camuti? Why didn't he call?

Then, suddenly, Balaban stood up and came out from under the dining table. He went into the kitchen and ate his breakfast. I followed him and hunkered down beside him trying to get a look at his eye. I called his name several times, hoping he would turn to me. But he ignored me completely. When he finished eating, he turned and went back under the dining table, tucked his front paws back into mandarin position, and that was it.

I breathed a little easier. It didn't seem to me that he could be in pain if he was eating. Therefore, he most likely was not going to go blind or lose an eye. I secretly cursed cats for being the mysterious creatures they are. If Balaban was a dog I might have known something instead of stringing suppositions together. And where was Camuti?

And come to think of it, who the hell was this Camuti that his name should just pop into my mind? I mentally went over the names of other cat owners among our friends to try to locate which one had first mentioned the legendary veterinarian? But I drew a blank.

Yet I had instinctively called for him knowing he was the man for our beloved cat. What did I know about him? Very little beyond the incredible fact that in this day and age he made house calls for cats, and that whenever his name came up in conversations, it was followed by an assortment of anecdotes attesting to Camuti as the miracle worker, the character, the curmudgeon.

The more I tried to put it all together in my mind, the more I came to the conclusion that Camuti just *was*. In the world of cat people, he was on a par with Morris the Cat, and Little Friskies and Litter Green—the names one accepted automatically without any adjectives required.

Maybe so, but the morning crept by without a return call from Dr. Camuti. Finally, at 1:37 P.M., the telephone rang. I picked it up and a gravelly voice said, "Camuti here."

"Thank God," I said and blurted out everything.

When I finished, Camuti—the way he referred to himself—said dryly, "But the cat is eating?"

"Yes."

"Doesn't sound too bad. I'll be by sometime in the evening."

"Evening!" I shouted, and then pulled my voice down. "Can't you come now?"

"I don't begin my rounds until late afternoon. If you want someone right away, you'd better . . ."

"No, no, I guess we can wait." Better to wait for a name I had heard of than to take Balaban to a complete stranger.

The doctor said, "Give me your address and apartment number. Are you in an elevator building? I'm no spring chicken anymore."

I assured him we had elevators.

11

The last thing he said before he hung up was, "I hope you have a bar of Ivory soap and some whiskey—preferably vodka —in the house. If not vodka, anything else will do. But definitely the Ivory."

"I'll get some," I said as the telephone connection was broken.

I hung up and confusion set in. I could understand the soap he washed up before or after examining a cat—but why the vodka? Did he drink? Had I waited all day to turn Balaban over to an alcoholic veterinarian?

The tension mounted in the room from 5:45 when Marilyn came home until 7:18—I checked my wristwatch—when Max rang up from the lobby. "There's a Dr. Cutie here." Max had never gotten a visitor's name right in the five years we had lived in the building.

"Send him up," I said.

Marilyn touched absent-mindedly at her hair. Eartha came in from the bathroom where he had been sleeping on the mat to sniff at Balaban under the table. Balaban didn't open his eyes as his brother poked at him with his nose.

And I stared at the door, waiting for the bell to ring. In my mind, I pictured Dr. Camuti looking like a cross between Robert Young as Marcus Welby and my dim childhood movie memories of Jean Hersholt as kindly old Dr. Christian.

Suddenly, there were two short, sharp rings from the apartment bell. Eartha shot out of the room. Balaban made a sad sound but didn't move. Marilyn and I nearly collided as we ran to the door.

The man in the doorway bore absolutely no resemblance to any television or movie doctor. He was short and wore a hat and coat. Beyond a portion of nose sticking out beneath his hat brim I couldn't see his face. But there was authority in his posture which had a military stiffness. "Frankel?" he said.

"Yes."

"Camuti." He brushed by us and entered the room. I cannot explain it to this day, but I became aware of it at our first meeting and have never lost sight of it since: Louis Camuti has a way of entering a room and immediately capturing it. It becomes his room, and the owners of the room—at least, this owner—feel like trespassers on their own ground.

He glanced around with the professional eye of an auctioneer making an appraisal, put his bag down on the dining table which my wife had long forbidden me to put anything on for fear of scratching it, took off his hat and unbuttoned his coat. He folded the coat neatly and put it over a chair.

He was bald and no beauty. His nose was the predominant feature on his face, that is until you noticed his eyes, which seemed to jump from object to object around the room. "Well, where's Oswilla?"

We both looked blank, not knowing what he was talking about.

"The patient," he said in his gravelly voice. I began to wonder if he ever spoke in lengthy sentences.

Then he chuckled, short and dry. The first warmth of his personality came through. "I can't remember every cat's name. I see so many of them. So I call all females Oswilla and all males Nicodemus."

"*His* name is Balaban and *he* is under the table," Marilyn said.

"Balaban? That's a new one on me," Camuti said. "I don't think I'll ever learn that one. Well, get him out and bring him into the kitchen while I scrub up. You've got the Ivory soap?"

"It's in the bathroom," Marilyn said. "This way, Doctor."

"Please bring it into the kitchen. I'd rather wash there," he said. "And bring the vodka or whatever along, too."

I crawled under the table. Balaban gave a sad little cry as I touched him, and tried to pull further into himself. I patted him on the head. "Nobody's going to hurt you, Bal. The doctor's going to make you better."

He cried again as I pulled him out from under the table. I carried him into the kitchen where Camuti was drying his hands on paper toweling. He took the cat from me and set him on the kitchen counter. "You got the vodka?" he said over his shoulder. Balaban hunched up and spat at him. Camuti chuckled. "That sounds pretty healthy to me. Now, let's see who socked you, Nicodemus."

13

I got down the vodka from the cabinet over the refrigerator. Marilyn was standing just outside of the kitchen, jamming the knuckles of her left hand against her mouth. There were tears running down her cheeks.

"I want you to hold him firmly while I take a look at his eye," Camuti said.

I placed my hands on either side of Balaban. "Hang onto him," the doctor said. "I'm not going to hurt him, but he doesn't know that."

Balaban spit and hissed as the doctor gently opened his eye. Camuti laughed. "That's it, Nicodemus. Give 'em hell."

He released the cat's head. Balaban spat again. "Do you people have any other cats or dogs?"

"Yes, Eartha. That's Balaban's brother. Did he do that to him?"

"Probably, if that's the only other animal you've got." He opened his bag. "I need some tissues or toilet paper. And open the vodka bottle."

Marilyn ran to the bathroom for the tissue box.

"Well, we go to the country weekends," I said, "and we do let the cats outdoors."

"Then it could have been anything. I'll tell you this, it happened about two days ago. Just a minor scratch."

Marilyn brought in the tissues and opened the vodka.

"Keep holding him," Camuti said. "Don't worry. You won't break him." He uncapped a disposable hypodermic syringe. "I'm going to give him an antibiotic shot, and we'll put some ointment in that eye to soothe the inflammation. You'll have to put the ointment in twice a day for the next few days."

I groaned. He looked at me and smiled. "What's the matter? You're bigger than the cat. I'll show you how."

He took some tissues and wadded them, then soaked them with vodka. "Good drinking," he said, "but a better antiseptic." So much for his drinking problem.

He wiped a patch of Balaban's fur with the vodka. Before Balaban could swing his head to get at Camuti's hand, I saw Camuti's arm flash through the air in a blur. Balaban got his shot.

14

Camuti winked at me. "Did you even see it? Louis Camuti, the fastest shot in the East."

He opened a small tube of ointment. "Now, pay attention, young man, and we'll make a veterinarian of you yet."

I grunted. He took hold of Balaban under the chin. "First thing is you get a firm grip on the cat."

To my amazement, he began putting the salve in the wrong eye. "Doctor! That's not the eye."

He nodded. "I know. I'm just confusing the cat. They have a tendency to rub at the eye you treat. By treating both eyes, I mix him up and the ointment stays in longer and does more good." I looked at Marilyn. There was respect in her eyes, too. "Okay, you can let him go now."

Balaban leaped from the table and shot out of the kitchen and into our bedroom where I assume he went under the bed. Camuti handed the tube of salve to me. "Twice a day. Once in the morning and once at night."

He closed the bag. I led the way into the living room. Marilyn said, "Can I get you something? Would you care to sit down?"

"No to both," he said, rocking slightly on his feet. "I'm like a horse. I rest standing up. Maybe that's why I've lasted so long."

He could tell we didn't know to what he was referring. "You know how old I am? I'm eighty-five, what do you think of that?" He looked from Marilyn to me. We were both amazed. He looked like a man in his sixties.

He reminded me of a rooster, the short fighting-cock type. His flamboyant necktie—it looked like someone had spilled plums down his shirt front—enhanced the image. Mostly it was the way he moved. Short swift gestures. He didn't swing his head when he looked from me to Marilyn. Instead, he seemed to snap it, cocking it slightly along the way. And he continued to rock on his feet.

Each time Camuti rocked back on his heels there was a strange sound, like tiny beads rolling against each other far away. Marilyn and I looked at each other. "What is that?" she asked.

Camuti gave his dry laugh and reached into his jacket pocket.

He pulled out something made of crystal with silver at both ends. "Pills."

The container was packed. "You take all of those?" I asked.

He shook his head. "Some are for cats, and some are for their owners. The rest are for me. I'm allergic to cats."

Having tossed that minor bombshell, he picked up his bag and started for the door. I helped him on with his coat. "Nicodemus should be a brand-new cat by tomorrow morning," he said, "but keep up with that salve for at least the next two days."

We nodded. Marilyn asked, "Will you want to see him again?"

"I'll stop by on Wednesday evening and have a look."

We nodded again. At the door, I said, "What days do you make rounds, Doctor? I mean just in case we need you again."

He cocked his head to look at me from under the brim of his hat. "Let's not go so fast, young man. We can discuss that on Wednesday after I see Nicodemus."

"What do you mean?"

He turned in the doorway to face us both. "I'm not saying you are, and I'm not saying you're not my clients yet. That depends. I have three rules. First, you have to love your pet and care for it. Second, you have to follow my instructions. And third, you have to pay your bills on time. I'll know the answer to the first two on Wednesday, and we'll see about the third on the first of the month."

He tipped his hat to Marilyn, turned smartly and headed for the elevator, never looking back.

When the door was closed, Marilyn said, "Isn't he something?"

I laughed. "But I think I like him."

"He's like eating snails. An acquired taste."

"More like an artichoke, I think. If you can get past the prickly choke, there's a lot of heart inside."

The next morning, Balaban's eye was half open, and he showed up along with his indifferent brother at the food bowls. It was at the first sight of the restored Balaban that our love affair with Dr. Louis J. Camuti began.

HF

16

Chapter I

I CANNOT TELL YOU how often I've been asked by a client, "Doctor, do you really like cats?" I usually just stare at the person who asks and say nothing. But to myself I think, "All of my clients are normal, but some are more normal than others." It's a favorite expression of mine, and the kindest way I can put it.

It has occurred to me that maybe the question has something to do with my catside manner. I admit that I am not always the most charming man in the world, but I don't think I am too bad. I grant you that I could be warmer and more soothing to an anxious pet owner if I had more time. But usually, when Alex —my wife, Alexandra—and I start off on my nightly rounds driving through the streets of New York City, I have a full schedule of patients waiting for me.

What I really want to say to the person who asks me that question is: "I've been practicing veterinary medicine since January of 1920, and most of that time has been spent with cats. Now, can you tell me any reason why a man—assuming he's not a maniac—would spend nearly sixty years of his life attending to animals he doesn't like?"

Frankly, I don't think the question has anything to do with me. It has to do with cat people, not all of them, but a lot of them. I doubt if veterinarians who take care of dogs or parakeets or even kangaroos ever get asked that question. It's not that dog or parakeet—I don't really know that much about kangaroos—people love their pets any the less, it's just that they don't seem to go crazy the way some cat owners I've known do.

Yes, of course, I like cats. I can only say love in terms of my own cats, when I had them. Love, I think, can only exist between the owner and his or her cat. But I like them. If I didn't, I would do something else for a living.

I certainly don't like all cats. Some of my patients are downright vicious. But most of them are just fine and highly likable—though it's a rare cat that has liked me when I was its doctor—and there are several that I saw often enough to become very fond of. But by and large, I think I feel about my patients the way a general practitioner feels about his or hers. A person or an animal in pain reaches out for your heart, and you want to help to relieve the pain. A doctor supplies his talent; it's the owner who supplies the love.

I seem to have made a pretty big deal about cats and love, so I think it's time to tell about the first cat in my life, and one I loved very much. I remember everything about her except how she came to be named Ci-Nin. She was the cat that saved my life when I was just a kid, maybe ten or eleven years old.

My father and mother, my younger brother, Joseph Louis, and I—I'm Louis Joseph—arrived in this country from Parma, Italy, on March 17, 1902, when I was nine years old. Our first home was an apartment at 104 MacDougal Street in Greenwich Village. We didn't live there too long because my father decided it was crazy to bring the whole family halfway across the world to settle in an Italian neighborhood. So he moved us up to Leland Avenue in the Upper Bronx, which tonier people said was Westchester.

But before we left MacDougal Street, Ci-Nin came into our lives, thanks to my mother. My mother was a loving and religious woman. I think she loved everything on God's green earth, but she especially loved animals. Mama had only to step out of our apartment to meet an animal somewhere that caught at her heart. It could be a hungry kitten in front of the fish store, or some pigeons on the corner of Sixth Avenue, or a dog that seemed lost in the street. Before Mama came home, the kitten had fish scraps from the store owner, the pigeons got cookie or bread crumbs from her shopping basket, and the dog found a home with someone on the block. That was Mama's way. The minute she saw an animal in need, tears came into her eyes and she went into action.

I can still see my mother sitting by the window that looked out onto the street and shelling peas into a bowl. Suddenly, she leaped up, told me to watch my younger brother until she came back. She ran from the apartment while I rushed to the window dragging Joseph with me. The poor kid wasn't tall enough to see over the window sill.

I saw Mama rush into the street and up to a man who was beating the horse that pulled his wagon. I don't know what Mama said, but I saw her grab the leather strap from the man's hand and start shaking it in his face. Mama was a tiny woman, and the man was huge and towered over her. He could have brushed her off the street with the back of his hand but he never had a chance. Mama was shouting and waving the strap at him as if she was going to whale the tar out of him at any second. The poor guy just stood pressed with his back against his cart until Mama finished everything she had to say. Then with a dramatic gesture, she flung the strap at him and turned grandly and marched back toward our house. The strap fell to the street; the man just stood there in shock.

When Mama returned, she gathered my brother and me in front of her. "Did you see that?" she asked.

I said I did, and Joseph, who hadn't seen anything, nodded, too. "I want you both to remember this always," she said, raising a finger in front of our faces to drive the lesson home, "God made people and he made animals. He meant for them to live in peace with each other. One is not better than the other. The strong should take care of the weak. To hurt an animal or a person that has not hurt you is cruel. And it is a sin. Don't ever let me catch either of you hurting an animal that has not hurt you."

We promised.

And that was the reason why my brother and I rushed into the middle of a gang of boys who were tossing a dirty little kitten around as if it were a baseball. Each time the kitten flailed its legs or made frightened noises the ruffians laughed.

I imagine that if the boys knew what had hit them they would have beat the stuffings out of me and Joseph. But we were a surprise commando raid. We grabbed the kitten and were gone before they even knew we were there.

We took it straight home to Mama and told her what had happened. She kissed us both and told us we could keep the kitten. The minute I put it down, the frightened animal dashed under the sofa, and didn't show its face again for two hours. Mama lured it out with a bit of hamburger meat on a saucer. But it was such a frightened animal that it only came out if no one was in the parlor, or if we sat very, very still and across the room.

No sooner did it eat than it ran back to its hiding place again. It took three days for Ci-Nin to become comfortable with the Camutis and come out to be with us.

She turned out to be a beauty, too, when she had gotten herself cleaned up. The dirty gray kitten we had brought home turned out to be all white with large orange eyes and a very loving nature.

I don't know why, since we all spoiled her and would slip her special treats under the dinner table—something I strongly advise my clients never to do—but I was Ci-Nin's favorite. Whenever I was home, Ci-Nin stayed close to me. She followed me from room to room, and she would curl up in my lap while I did my homework. And when it was time for bed, Ci-Nin leaped onto my bed and curled up for the night. I loved Ci-Nin, but the bedtime honors were something I could do without because Ci-Nin was a terrible bed hog.

When we moved up to Leland Avenue I hoped the different rooms would confuse Ci-Nin and she might not find my bed, but she was there from the first night, fighting me for the center of the bed, walking right up my body to stare into my face when she decided it was time for me to get up.

It was while we were living on Leland Avenue that I came down with typhoid fever, a dread disease in those days. None of the miracle drugs existed back then, so the treatment was bed rest—three solid months of it—and a bland liquid diet. I lost a great deal of weight and was so weak that I couldn't even turn my body in bed. My mother had to turn me from side to side to prevent bed sores. Even so, I got them.

If I wasn't so sick I probably would have gone out of my mind from boredom in those days before television and radio. I was too weak to read. My only distraction was Ci-Nin, who played all her cat games with me. Her favorite was catch-the-mouse-that's-under-the-covers, which meant that any time I wiggled a toe Ci-Nin attacked it.

Another favorite game of Ci-Nin's was trying to eat out of my bowl whenever my mother brought me soup on a tray. As far as Ci-Nin was concerned, my illness suited her just fine. Instead of being left alone all day while I was at school, Ci-Nin now had company around the clock.

One morning, my mother went across the hall to visit a neighbor for a few minutes, leaving Ci-Nin asleep on top of my bed. Either Mama forgot or she only expected to be gone for a few minutes because she left my lunch broth heating on top of the stove.

The liquid boiled away, and the beef started to burn against the side of the dry pot. Smoke began to fill the apartment. I became aware of a funny smell, but I was too weak and tired to open my eyes. I felt Ci-Nin walk up the bed. She pushed her face against mine and meowed. I pushed her away with my hand. Then I felt her rough, wet tongue on my neck and arm, but I couldn't bring myself out of my feverish sleep. I flopped a weak hand again to drive her away. Ci-Nin put her paw on my lips and pushed at them, never bringing out her claws, but I ignored her.

The smell was strong, cutting into my sleep, and I could feel Ci-Nin's activities becoming more agitated on my covers. Suddenly, my eyes popped open as Ci-Nin gave me a swat across the cheek. That woke me and I saw the room through a haze of blackish, acrid smoke. I began choking, and I realized what Ci-Nin had been trying to do.

I opened my mouth to call for help, but it only led to a coughing fit. I was certain I was going to die.

Miraculously, my mother came running into the room and threw open the windows. Then she ran back to turn off the stove.

When the air cleared I could see that the door to the bedroom down the hall was wide open. The smoke had to have been thinner in there, and Ci-Nin could have run there to save herself. Instead, she had stayed on top of the bed to help me at what might have been the cost of her own life.

Now, if you want to get technical about it, my mother saved my life. And you can say that the reason Ci-Nin kept trying to wake me was so that I could save her life, but that strikes me as pretty complex thinking for a cat. Anyway, I refuse to think of it that way. As far as I am concerned, Ci-Nin did everything a loving cat could do to save my life, and I will always remember her that way.

Often, I've been asked if I think Ci-Nin was the reason I became a veterinarian specializing in cats. My answer is either no or I don't know. And I'll tell you this, I don't go for any of that hogwash about Ci-Nin affecting my subconscious so that even not knowing it, I was destined to be a cat doctor.

Frankly, I think psychology and psychiatry are great for those people who need them and believe in them. I am from an earlier generation, one that didn't sit around and moan about what was done to us as kids and what we might have been if things were different. I can't worry about what might have been. I believe you take whatever you were given to work with, and you get up and get out and make the most of it. And that's what I've done.

I became a veterinarian specializing in cats because that was what I wanted to do with my life. And that's all there is to it as far as I know. I can't waste two minutes thinking about what might have been because I am completely satisfied with what I am.

Chapter 2

I SOMETIMES WONDER what other people whose work takes them all over New York City see when they look out their car windows. Does the accountant see the Seagram Building when he drives by or does he see just one window where his client, Mr. So-and-So, has his offices? Does the dentist see Central Park or does his mind go oh-oh, there's the bridle path where Mrs. Whosis lost her bridge when her horse reared? I wonder, because wherever Alex and I go on our nighttime rounds I see cats. Not buildings or people, but cats.

As I turn the corner onto a street that I don't think I've ever had a patient on before, suddenly a whiskery face pops in front of my eyes. Often I can't even remember the cat's name or who it belonged to, but when I see those big eyes looking at me from the sooty face of a Siamese or the orange, brown and white of a calico, I know I've been there before. For example, when I turn off Seventh Avenue into 41st Street and go past a theater they now call the Trafalgar, what I see is the old name National and then Barbara Baxley's cat, Tula. I suppose if I was to make up a map of New York City, there wouldn't be one famous landmark and very few street names. West 41st Street would be called Tula Street, and over on the East Side there would be Barnaby-and-Tulip Avenue for Phyllis Levy's cats. And down in the Village would be the-cat-belonging-to-the-nudist-at-the-piano alley.

I've sometimes wondered if Alexandra sees the city the way I do, since she has been driving around with me for so long now, but I've never asked her. If I know my Alex, she'd just make a gesture of dismissal with her hand and say, "Oh, Wrinks"—she gave me the nickname of Wrinkles years ago—and go ahead with whatever she was doing to pass the time while I was in with a patient.

You'd think that when a man of my years is still running around in the service of his patients, there'd be a little appreciation on their part for me. But out of the thousands of cats I have tended in my time, I'd really have to wrack my brain to come up with one who was ever glad to see me—or was even *there* to see me when I came through the door.

That's the worst part of my kind of medical practice. In any other medical specialty, when a doctor makes an appointment to see a patient they will both show up. But all I have to do is give my usual two short rings at an apartment door and my patient disappears. And when a cat decides to do a disappearing act, believe me it makes Judge Crater look like a piker. A cat determined to hide can find places even in a two-by-four, one-room apartment that the person paying the rent doesn't know exist. A cat determined not to be found can fold itself up like a pocket handkerchief if it wants to.

Because I'm usually running on a tight schedule when Alex and I set out for a night's work, I can't hang around an apartment waiting while the owners try to flush out their cat. That's why I've created what I call the Camuti System and taught it to clients whose cats require several visits from me. Ideally, I want my clients to put the patient in the bathroom and close the door so it can't take off when I ring the bell, but even in such tight quarters as the average New York City bathroom a couple of cats have outwitted me in their time. But if the cat is still running around when I show up, we have to put the Camuti Method into action. It's really very simple and logical and usually flushes out the patient. You begin at one end of the apartment and work your way to the other end, carefully checking out the first room, looking behind, and under everything a cat could possibly hide in. Then you close the door on that room, and proceed to search the next, again closing the door behind you before you move on to the third room. By all logic, you should have the cat by the time you hit the end of the apartment.

But not always. When Tom and Lois Wallace's Siamese, Rajah, got sick, the Wallaces, their young son, George, the maid and I went through the entire apartment with the Camuti Method and ended up without Rajah. Considering that Rajah was fifteen years old—hardly a spring chicken anymore—and a dignified Siamese at that, one wouldn't expect any high jinks from him. Some haughty Siamese yowling and hissing maybe, but not this.

Tom, Lois and I ended up in the kitchen scratching our heads, and catless. Little Georgie, their son, refused to give up and started through the apartment again. Aside from determination, Georgie also had the advantage of his youth and size in the search, and could look under things more easily than we could. That's what undid Rajah.

Georgie called his parents to come into their bedroom. I remained in the kitchen until I heard the whole family laughing. When I entered the bedroom, the three Wallaces were on their hands and knees beside the bed. Tom signaled me to join them. "Look what George spotted," Tom said, and pointed to a lump in the underside of the box spring just a little to the right of a rip in the covering. Tom reached out and gave a poke and the lump moved. Another poke, this time on the other side, so that, they hoped, the lump would move toward the rip and fall through. But Rajah was too smart for that. He moved forward, parallel to the rip. "I'll be damned," I said, mentally tipping my hat to Rajah for his ingenuity.

To get Rajah out, we had to fan out, three Wallaces at three corners and Camuti at the fourth, remove the mattress and then lift the box spring and tilt it back and forth as if we were panning for gold or jiggling a pinball machine. From inside the box spring came the weirdest collection of sounds as Rajah protested his treatment and tried to dig in. Finally, we outmaneuvered him and he fell through the hole and took his treatment. The Wallaces sewed up the box spring before my next visit. No one —with the possible exception of Rajah—was willing to go through that routine again.

I would have said Rajah was unique in his choice of hiding place if over the years I hadn't helped dig other cats out from other beds. Maybe it's their height that allows cats to see a rip that they can crawl into, or maybe their fear of Camuti inspires the cat to make the rip. Whatever it is, in my experience, cats and beds seem to be a natural combination.

Miss Livingston's cat, a pale-gray shorthair named Mopsy, was another bed hider. Miss Livingston, an executive secretary in the Wall Street area, had a very tidy four-room apartment that she shared with Mopsy and Mopsy's brother, Topsy. Because she had to work late and didn't want to delay the cats' yearly shots, she left the keys to the apartment for me with the door-man. When I entered, I found only Topsy, who got his shot. Though I searched the apartment from stem to stern there was no Mopsy. I left a note for Miss Livingston to find Mopsy and put her in the bathroom before my next visit.

When the time came, I found Miss Livingston waiting for me in the hall in front of her door. She put a finger across her lips to silence me. "What are you doing out here?" I whispered.

"I don't want you to ring the bell," she said. "Mopsy knows your ring. Wait till you see where she hides."

I had a long night ahead of me and I wasn't in the mood for cat games. "In the mattress," I said.

Miss Livingston looked at me, surprised, and said, "You're right, but wait until you see how."

She signaled me to follow her. Then she opened the door noisily and said loudly, "Come in, Dr. Camuti."

I saw Topsy duck under the sofa, but it was Mopsy who really caught my eye. The cat was no more than a gray blur as it shot in front of us and headed toward the back of the apartment. Miss Livingston said, "Come quickly and watch."

If there was an Olympics for cats, Mopsy could have taken a

gold medal for gymnastics. She shot down the hall, took a hairpin turn past the bathroom, somehow bounced herself off the bedroom door and shot across about three feet of open air and into a flap in the side of the mattress. My eyes were still taking it all in as the gray tail disappeared, as if it were being sucked up into the mattress.

Mopsy looked very sulky when I reached in and pulled her out and gave her her shot. I couldn't blame her. She deserved applause, not an injection.

A cat owner suffers more than his pet when a cat gets an injection. It's all that hissing, spitting and struggling that convinces the owner his cat is in agony. The truth is that the injections are normally not very painful. The intensity of the pain depends on many factors:

1. The sharper the needle, the less pain there is. The disposables we use today keep needle pain to a minimum.

2. The pain varies with the type of medication. Thiamin (B_1) is more painful than most other injections.

3. The seat of injection makes a difference. Subcutaneous injections are the least painful.

4. Intravenous injections cause varying degrees of pain.

5. The faster you inject, the shorter the traumatic period.

Because I have grown so accustomed to finding cats in or under beds, when all else fails I start poking around mattresses. The bedroom search got me one hell of a surprise at Margaret Sangster's house. She was a very successful writer of radio soap operas. Usually when I arrived I'd find Miss Sangster in the middle of her work with three secretaries helping her. One would be taking dictation, a second would be transcribing dictation, and the third would be putting the transcriptions into proper script form. She and I would just wave to each other and she would point to the stairs, meaning the cat was up in her bedroom waiting for me.

Though I didn't know it, the day I'm thinking of was the day following one of her famous parties. Margaret Sangster's parties always started out like normal parties, but what made them famous was Margaret's attitude, which was easy and casual. She was a generous woman with food and drink, and she had a full staff to see to her guests, and all her friends knew it. Very often, an evening planned for twenty grew to forty or more as each friend brought along a couple of his or her friends.

Naturally, when I opened her bedroom door I didn't see the cat, so I closed the door behind me and began to search the room. Based on past experiences, the first thing I did was to get down on my hands and knees and look under the bed. What I saw made me rear up and smack my noggin on the mattress frame. There was a woman's body, fully dressed, under there.

I didn't know if the woman was dead or alive as I headed for the stairs and straight down to where Margaret and her secretaries were working. "Margaret, there's a body under your bed," I blurted out.

The three secretaries froze. Margaret just looked at me with mild impatience, as if I had interrupted her work to tell her it was raining outside. "That's impossible, Louie. I slept there all night."

"Well, whether you slept there or not, it's up there."

Margaret gave some orders to her secretaries, put down the papers she was holding and followed me up the stairs. We both got down on the floor beside the bed and looked. "Is she alive?" Margaret asked.

I reached out and felt the woman's wrist. "Yes."

Margaret stood up and brushed at her skirt. "Well, I don't know her," she said. "She must be left over from the party."

Margaret excused herself and went back to her work. Obviously, she considered the matter closed. Being under the bed was the woman's problem, not Margaret Sangster's.

Well, it certainly wasn't mine, so I continued my search for the cat, which I found squeezed in behind a bureau. When I left the bedroom, the cat had been tended to and the woman was still asleep under the bed. When she came out I have no idea. For all I know, Margaret Sangster had her butler slide trays under the bed three times a day. She and I never talked about the incident again.

Minor Latham's ginger cat, Singer, was another bed hider, which was usually where I found her—Singer, not Miss Latham —because no matter how many times I told her, Miss Latham never seemed to remember to lock up the cat when I was expected. But I'd bet that was about the only thing Miss Latham forgot.

Red-haired and frisky and probably in her seventies, Minor Latham was a member of the English Department of Barnard College before World War One and became head of the department in the 1930s. After she retired in 1948, Barnard named a theater in her honor because she had also taught drama there. Though she rarely looked back and reminisced—"There's too much to do tomorrow," she once said—she once told me that Jane Wyatt, Aline MacMahon and Helen Gahagan Douglas had been students of hers.

After her retirement, she continued to live within walking distance of Columbia and Barnard. She had a four-bedroom apartment on Claremont Avenue. If that sounds like too large a place for a single lady, one cat and a live-in maid, you don't know Minor Latham. She hung onto anything and everything that her mother, father, grandparents and friends had ever collected. Most of the stuff was under one bed or another, and considering that she had two beds in each of her four bedrooms, you can picture how much she had in that apartment. But despite it all, the place was always in apple-pie order when I paid a visit, and the maid always looked nervous and exhausted, which told me that Minor Latham ran a tight ship. In fact, though her maid had been with her for twenty years at the time I knew Miss Latham, she never called the woman by name. Whenever she wanted anything, she just shouted "Maid!" and the poor woman came running.

But I liked Minor Latham—I've always been drawn to characters—except for her continuously forgetting to trap Singer in the bathroom before I showed up.

The visit I'm thinking of took place around 10 P.M. on a rainy night. I was tired and wet, and all I wanted to do was get home and put my feet up. I prayed that just this once Miss Latham would remember and have Singer waiting for me in the bathroom. But, as usual, she hadn't, so we began the Camuti Method search, room by room, and bed by bed—all eight of them. By the time we got to the last bed in the last bedroom my knees were sore from all that bending and poking around among the boxes and bags under each bed.

I groaned out loud as I got down on my knees to look under the bed; I wanted Miss Latham to know I was annoyed with her —not that it would do any good. Suddenly I saw some ginger-colored fluff move way under the bed. At last! I reached out and grabbed and got a good hold. "Come out of there, you little so-and-so!"

To my amazement, I heard a scream instead of a yowl. It was Miss Latham on the other side of the bed. "Let go! Let go! You've grabbed my hair."

That did it. We gave up, and I went home. The next night Miss Latham telephoned to tell me that after I'd left she found the cat sitting in the middle of the living room. She ended the conversation with "I want you to know my head still hurts."

There was a young man whose name I can no longer remember, but I do know he had a new black kitten he wanted me to examine. He lived in a studio apartment at 57th Street and Sixth Avenue. Considering the size of the apartment and how sparsely it was furnished, you'd think you could find a missing pin, much less a kitten, the minute you entered. All he had was a mattress on the floor, and a few chairs around a wrought-iron table with a glass top. The room was a small square with no odd corners or nooks. There were two doors, one to a bathroom, the other to a closet, and neither of them had a cat behind it. The kitchen equipment was all flush with the wall in one corner so nothing could get behind the stove or refrigerator.

Since there didn't seem to be any place his kitten could be hiding, I cocked an eye at the man. "You sure you've got a cat?"

"Oh, yes," he assured me. "Her name is Louella."

"Well, you'd better get her out here, son. I can't stand around here all night."

He thought a minute. "I know what will get her. I'll open the refrigerator and take out some hamburger. She loves it. That'll bring her right away, you'll see."

It brought Louella faster than either of us expected. The minute he opened the refrigerator door, the kitten leaped out, shook her fur and seemed none the worse for the cold storage. Luckily, the young man had fed her only a half hour before I arrived, which had to be when the cat had gotten inside.

In all my years of looking for my patients, there is one cat disappearance I will never solve. And it happened right in my own house.

It began with a request from a friend of mine, Dr. Victor Carabba, to spay his cat. I had met Victor when we were both students in veterinary school, though he later switched to human medicine and became a very fine surgeon.

"You're crazy, Victor," I said, "do it yourself. You're a top surgeon and also a trained veterinarian."

"No, Louie," he said. "I'll be right over, and I'd rather you do it."

He showed up on our doorstep within the hour and presented me with a Siamese kitten I judged to be about six months old. The kitten was wriggling to get out of his grip.

"I still don't see why you won't do it yourself," I said, though I suspected the answer.

He blushed. "I just couldn't. If anything went wrong I couldn't face my children. But don't you worry if something should happen. She's still new to the family and the kids aren't that attached to her yet." With that, he left. I went to work. This was back in the days when the anesthesia we used might take twenty to thirty hours to wear off, and you had to turn the animal every hour so its lungs wouldn't fill up with fluid. Because of the anesthesia and the turning, I put the kitten in the shower stall of the bathroom next to our bedroom so I wouldn't have to go downstairs when it was time to turn her.

When Alex awakened in the morning, she took the sleeping kitten downstairs where she could watch it so I could sleep uninterrupted.

When I got up, I went down to the kitchen, where I found my wife and my mother-in-law, who was living with us, in a state of panic.

"What's the matter?" I asked.

"The cat," she said. "It's missing."

Alex told me that she put the cat down on paper toweling in the middle of the kitchen table while she and her mother had breakfast in the dining room. When they returned to the kitchen—"It was only about fifteen minutes, Wrinks"—the cat had vanished.

"Assuming she came to," I said, "she couldn't have gone very far. She'd still be pretty woozy."

Alex said they had searched the entire downstairs and come up with nothing.

At that moment, the telephone rang. It was Victor Carabba inquiring about his kitten. I told him the truth, and he said not to worry. He was sure the kitten would turn up at any minute. That made me feel a little better, but I'm not certain that Victor believed what he had said because he called me every fifteen minutes to find out if we had found the cat.

Alex, my mother-in-law and I began a step-by-step search of the kitchen. The kitten had to be in that room because Alex, doctor's wife that she is, knew to close all doors behind her when she went in to breakfast.

In desperation, I called a local moving company and asked them to send two big guys over to move our refrigerator. It was the last place left where the kitten could possibly be.

They got the refrigerator out about a foot from the wall. I told them to stop and I took a look. All that there was behind the refrigerator was dust, and there wasn't a single paw print in it.

Before I called Con Edison to move the stove, I got a flashlight and lay down on the floor to look. No kitten.

When it was time for Alex and me to start on our patient rounds, my mother-in-law swore to us that she wouldn't leave the kitchen for anything short of a national emergency. When the kitten showed up—it had to eat sometime!—she'd be there and she would tell us where it had hidden.

While we were gone, my son Louis, Jr., and his wife, Grace, came over. When they learned what had happened, Louis came up with his own solution. "Our cat Olney hates all other cats. I'll bring him right over. He'll sniff out that kitten one-two-three."

Olney arrived and went crazy in the kitchen, clawing, hissing and screaming. But that's all my son's crazy cat did. Finally, Louis had to grab Olney and put him in his carrier. Unfortunately, my mother-in-law followed Louis and Grace to the front hall where he had left Olney's carrier. Once out of the kitchen Olney calmed down.

Louis went back to the kitchen to wash his hands. He let out a yip of surprise. There was Victor Carabba's kitten sitting calmly in the middle of the floor cleaning its fur.

That evening, I took the kitten straight to the Carabba house.

To this day, whenever I think of the kitten that pulled a Houdini on Camuti I look suspiciously all around our kitchen, trying to figure out a spot that Alex and I might have overlooked. We never have figured out where it could have hidden itself, and I am still tempted to have Con Edison come over and move our stove. If I could find just one cat hair behind it, I would be a happy man.

Chapter 3

MY ALLERGIES aren't one bit funny to me, but I can tell from the way people react—a faint smile that they quickly cover with a coughing attack, or an exaggerated "Oh, really? How interesting!"—that there is something humorous in the idea of a veterinarian being allergic to cats and dogs. As a friend of mine put it, "You've got to admit, Louie, it's like a fat Weight Watchers instructor, or a window washer who can't take heights." Well, I guess so, but here I am, an allergic cat doctor.

I first became aware of the problem in 1961 thanks to Toppolina II who liked to watch television sitting on my lap. Toppolina II was a dachshund puppy—dachsies are great favorites of mine. It happened one night when she jumped off my lap, and I felt a hot spot on my wrist where the puppy had been nuzzling. I looked, and there was a red blotch on my skin. At first I didn't pay any attention to the spot, but it happened again the next night. I realized that wherever Toppolina touched me or even breathed on me there'd be another red blotch that turned into a fiery rash.

I called my doctor and the next thing I knew I was in Doctors Hospital in Manhattan. I was told it was the only way they could isolate me from the source or sources of my rash while they ran tests on me to determine the cause. Not that there was much doubt. Poor Toppolina. I loved that little dachsie and now she was going to have to find a new home again. She was really leading a dog's life.

Toppolina II came to us through a lovely lady named Snow Viles. Mrs. Viles originally owned a dachshund named Nico, as well as a male Siamese cat. The Siamese had no real name because he wouldn't answer to one, according to Snow and Jimmy Viles. He only came if Mrs. Viles called out, "Siamese" or her husband's name, "Jimmy."

Siamese tolerated Nico, but no other animal. To be blunt, Siamese was a tough customer. Out at the Viles's summer place on Fire Island, Siamese patrolled the garden and kept it free of any and all animal intruders. In the city, he watched over the apartment with the same ferocity. You could usually find him perched on some high piece of furniture, ready to pounce on anything with four legs that came into the apartment.

When Nico died, Snow Viles got herself a new dachshund pup—the cat was really her husband's pet.

She telephoned me and asked me to come and examine the dachsie. I thought she was the cutest I'd ever seen. Because Alex and I had recently lost our own beloved Toppolina, I asked Mrs. Viles if she would mind bringing her puppy out to the car. I knew Alex would love it.

Alex oohed and aahed as I knew she would. I don't know for certain whether or not she meant it or was just making polite conversation, but Alex said, "If you ever decide to give her away she can come to us."

Mrs. Viles just laughed. Who would give away such a beautiful little dachsie? She had warm melting eyes and a coat the color of dark honey.

But about two weeks later, Mrs. Viles telephoned. "The dog is yours." The way she said it there was no doubting that she meant it.

I started to tell her that ours hadn't really been a serious offer. She cut me off. "The cat is trying to kill it."

As best as either of the Vileses could figure out, Siamese was convinced the puppy was a rat. He spent all day stalking the puppy from on high. Then he would pounce, grab it by the scruff of the neck and shake it, trying to break its neck. Keeping an eye on the cat and the puppy all day was just too much for Mrs. Viles, and no matter how hard she and her husband tried they just couldn't seem to keep them separated. The new dog simply had to go. Alex and I gave in with almost no struggle.

We rechristened her Toppolina II in memory of our first dachsie and fell hopelessly in love with her. As a veterinarian, I probably know better than most dog owners what is inside the animal's coat, but as far as I am concerned, inside Toppolina's coat there was just one big loving heart. In no time at all, little Toppolina II became a part of the Camuti household and adjusted to our strange hours. Watching television with me became a part of the dog's nightly routine, and that's when I started to itch.

I knew the experts at Doctors Hospital were going to tell me that I was allergic to dogs, but I was sunk when they said I was also allergic to cats, most other animals, dust, fungi and dozens of other things. What was going to happen to my practice, my patients, my whole livelihood? I was sixty-seven, too old to start a new career, but not old enough to retire my shingle.

Luckily, the doctors told me that they could control my allergy to cats and dogs for about twelve hours a day with antihistamines. That was fine for my professional life, but it meant that Alex and I could never have our own pets again. I thought of poor Toppolina II and when everyone had left the room I cried like a baby. But we found a good home for Toppolina II with friends in New Jersey where she lived a happy life.

That night in my hospital bed with the lights out and the tears running down my face in the dark, I thought of all the dogs and cats that had shared their lives with Alex and me. Each one was a special memory.

One of our favorites came to us in 1937 when we had just moved into our home in Westchester. One morning around eight o'clock, our son, Louis, who was ten at the time, came running into our bedroom and woke us up with the announcement that there was a cat with a big hernia on the back porch.

I groaned and begged Louis to let me sleep. I promised I would get up soon and look after the cat. That satisfied him for awhile, but not long enough for me to get the sleep I needed.

He was back in twenty minutes announcing new medical information at the top of his voice. It wasn't a hernia at all. That cat had given birth to five kittens on our porch. And what was I going to do about it?

Still groggy, I told him we could keep the mother if she didn't belong to a neighbor, but he would have to find homes for the five kittens. I thought that would keep him away from home long enough for me to get more sleep.

But Louis was back within an hour. He had found homes for all five kittens. I gave up and got out of bed.

Louis led me out to the porch where there were indeed five newborn kittens. The mother whom I had told Louis we would keep if she didn't belong to a neighbor was no beauty. One look and you knew she had lived a tough life on the streets. She was a broken-down swaybacked old scrapper that not even motherhood could give a warm and gentle look. But a deal was a deal.

I went back into the kitchen and poured myself a cup of coffee. Louis was jumping around, talking about the new cat and how much our Siamese, Chi-Chi, was going to love having a cat friend. Knowing Chi-Chi, who was definitely master of the house and had never let another animal enter, I strongly doubted it.

I made Louis sit quietly until I had gotten enough coffee inside me to feel awake. Then I asked the question that had been bothering me: How had Louis managed to find homes for five kittens in such a short time?

He told me it was easy. He had told everyone that if they took a kitten his father would neuter it at the right age and give it all of its necessary shots free.

"That was good thinking, son," I said a little sourly.

Louis swelled with pride.

As soon as they were old enough, each kitten went to its new home. And each kitten was brought back at the proper time. I spayed four females, and altered one male. Free!

I also spayed the mother of the brood before she presented us with another litter of freeloaders. We named her Mae West in tribute to the curvaceous movie star.

It was a good thing that we gave Mae West a home, because I doubt that we could have found one for her. Aside from being no beauty to look at, Mae lacked a heart-warming personality. She was a very aggressive street fighter, afraid of nothing on earth. Considering that she had been homeless all of her life, her lack of trust and charm was understandable.

Surprisingly enough, Mae West and Chi-Chi got along pretty well. I don't mean they got along together, but their living habits complimented each other's. Chi-Chi refused to share the house with another cat, and that suited Mae West just fine. She had lived her whole life out of doors and that was where she wanted to stay. Mae came around to the back porch for meals and took naps in the yard. She knew she belonged to a family but she still had the illusion that she was a free agent in the world.

The arrangement suited all of the Camutis through Mae's first spring and summer with us, but we weren't happy as the days grew shorter and colder. Tough and homely as the lady was, we had grown to love her and we wanted to bring her indoors for the winter. Mae seemed agreeable, and we hoped that after a squabble or two, she and Chi-Chi would learn to at least tolerate each other.

And so Mae West came indoors and the battles with Chi-Chi started. They went on day after day with neither cat giving an inch. There wasn't a night that we didn't come home to find clumps of fur somewhere in the house, evidence of another fight.

And then suddenly, peace reigned. The cats had worked it out between them. Chi-Chi retained control of the house, but Mae was mistress of the kitchen. They would occasionally trespass into each other's territory with much hissing, spitting and arching of backs, but it rarely came to claw-swinging blows.

The two battlers grew old together in separate parts of our house. The years went hissing and spitting by, and then Mae West developed a malignant growth on her jaw. I had to move her to my hospital, and when her discomfort became too great she was put to sleep.

Until the day Chi-Chi died, he rarely went into the kitchen. I like to think it was Chi-Chi's tribute to another fighter like himself. There is no doubt in my mind that Chi-Chi knew Mae West was gone.

Though my doctors had told me that my pet-keeping days were over, my clients weren't ready for me to give up on theirs. They didn't even wait until I got out of the hospital. The minute they found out that I was fit, they saw no reason why I should just lie there doing nothing, not when their animals needed me. That hospitals have rules forbidding pets didn't seem to stop my more determined clients.

Mary Henle was the first. She hadn't fought her way up the academic ladder to a full professorship of the New School just to be stopped by a mere hospital. Mary's cat, Guapo, a tough old customer, considering his age, had been seeing me three times every week for his geriatric shots. Treatment had begun when Guapo was fourteen years old—he was to live to the very ripe old age of twenty-one and a half years!—and Mary had no intention of losing him just because a hospital was being stuffy about animals.

I told Alex to tell Mary to come ahead, and when Dr. Nathan Kwit, my cardiologist, came to visit me, I asked him if he had a syringe in his bag that he could spare me. Needless to say, I didn't tell him about Guapo.

"What do you want with a syringe?" he asked.

"Oh, I just like to have one around. It helps me to remember that I still have a function in the outside world." It was the best I could come up with at the moment, and I saw Dr. Kwit looking at me in a funny way. So I added, "Maybe it's the allergy shots making me punchy. Anyway, I'd really like to have one."

He gave me a syringe from his black bag, and left shaking his head about poor old Louis Camuti.

Meanwhile, Mary had spoken with Alex, who arranged to meet her in the lobby about the time that visiting hours would be ending. I think the idea was that the mobs of visitors flowing out through the lobby might keep Mary and Guapo from being noticed.

Not that Mary's plan was as simple as that. Oh, no. Mary involved her twin sister, Jane, a professor of archeology. Though what Jane was supposed to do never became clear since the entire plan went awry the minute the women came through the hospital revolving door.

Mary had Guapo in a pillowcase, and he didn't like it one bit. The minute the ladies entered the lobby Guapo started crying on a rising note that threatened to turn into outraged yowling. Unfortunately, the cat's crying coincided with a sudden quiet in the lobby. To cover the sound, Jane started a noisy coughing fit, standing dead center in the middle of the lobby. Mary, meanwhile, raced over to Alex who was near the elevators. Alex rushed Mary and her now-howling pillowcase into an elevator. Once the doors closed behind them, Mary opened the pillowcase enough so Guapo could see her. It helped to quiet the terrified and angry cat.

Alex brought Mary to my room on a run. Guapo was starting his crying again. I figured we had only seconds before Guapo brought someone to my room to check on the strange sounds. Since Alex had brought my bag to the hospital during the afternoon, I loaded my syringe. I didn't even tell Mary to take Guapo out of the pillowcase. Instead, I just felt for his hind leg, and whammo! There was an angry yowl from inside, and I knew I had scored.

Alex meanwhile had gone out to the elevators and had one ready and waiting as Mary came running down the hall. But when they got to the lobby again—and now Mary didn't care if anyone heard Guapo or not—there was no Jane. They waited for ten minutes without a sign of Mary's twin sister. Finally Alex went to the visitor's desk, pointed out Mary and asked if the young man behind the desk had seen a woman who looked just like her.

Just then Jane showed up looking slightly frazzled. It turned out that she had done too good a job on her coughing fit, and two interns had grabbed her and taken her to Emergency over her protests. It was just as well, as Jane's bravura performance had caused her to irritate her throat.

I don't think it was Guapo's crying and yowling that gave me away to the hospital staff, but word did get around that there was a cat doctor in the house. Doctors, nurses and interns started dropping in just to see how I was getting along. At first, I thought it was just my charm that was drawing them. Then I became aware that every visit suddenly took a turn to, "By the way, I have this cat and I wonder . . ."

Everyone at the hospital who owned a cat wanted advice or just to talk about his or her cat. Still in bed and a patient, I found myself conducting a fairly active practice though it was mostly advice. That is, until a supervisor sneaked her cat in to see me. And then a nurse did the same thing. It made me feel better about Mary Henle's visit.

Then, one afternoon, the telephone by my bed rang. I picked it up and heard the no-nonsense voice of General Schwengel, a client of mine. He sounded very annoyed with me for daring to be in the hospital. "It's time for Kitty's stitches to come out!" he barked.

He was right, of course. I had spayed Miss Kitty, his Siamese, just before I had checked into Doctors Hospital. "General," I said, "I have a very good veterinarian covering for me while I'm in here. He can easily take out Miss Kitty's stitches."

"Won't do!" General Schwengel said flatly. "It has to be you. You're her doctor."

I laughed. "Then come ahead," I said, "if you think you can get your cat in here."

42

"We'll be there," he said and the telephone went dead.

I didn't have a doubt in my mind that General Schwengel and Miss Kitty would appear. General Schwengel was an artillery man from World War I, and there was no fooling with him. After he retired from the army in 1936 with the rank of brigadier general, he entered the business world. At the time that he became my client he was the retired chairman of Seagrams Distillers. He was obviously a man used to taking charge of any and all situations. Doctors Hospital didn't stand a chance.

I knew that he wouldn't come up with any plan such as Mary Henle tried to pull off. General Schwengel was a man who took direct action, which was exactly what he did.

He arrived at Doctors Hospital with Miss Kitty in her cat carrier being held by the Schwengels' cook and went straight up to the information desk and demanded my room number. The girl gave him the number, and then spotted the carrier. "But what are you doing with that, sir? You can't bring animals in here."

The General ignored her, signaled to his cook to come ahead, and marched straight to the elevators, leaving the woman at the information desk going, "But . . . but . . . but . . ." like an outboard motor.

"What the hell kind of hospital do they run around here?" he asked as he came through my door.

I removed the stitches with the help of one of the floor nurses who supplied me with scissors, tweezers and alcohol. Through the whole very simple procedure, the General stood stiff as starch beside his cat, crooning, "Good kitty, the doctor's not hurting you, that's a kitty, oh what a brave kitty."

When I had finished, Miss Kitty went back into her carrier, the General signaled the cook to pick it up, and off they marched, the General wearing that look of his that dared anyone to get in his way.

Within a few days, word got around the hospital about the General's visit. Dr. John Prutting, my internist, laughed it off—he never knew about Mary's visit—but he didn't think it was very funny when he heard that I was also seeing half of the cats belonging to hospital staff members.

"What's so wrong?" I said to him. "I'm paying a king's ransom for this private room, and I'm bored to tears. I've got a pretty nurse whenever I need an assistant, and you've got all the equipment I need."

"That isn't exactly how I see it," he said.

"Well, look at it this way," I said. "I'm giving away a fortune in office-visit fees. I could pay for this room and even make a profit if I started charging."

That did it. The next morning, Dr. Prutting sent me home.

Chapter 4

ONE GOOD THING—maybe the only good thing—about getting way up there in the eighties is that you know what's important in life. Or if you don't, you should at least know what's unimportant. Maybe that's why I didn't get too upset in the 1960s when the kids seemed to be taking over the whole world, saying get rid of this and get rid of that, it's all wrong and what does life really mean anyway?

I knew it all had to pass. Not because I'm so much brighter than anyone else. Anybody who's been around for a long time knows that just about everything passes with time and that what seems new today has probably been around before. And sure enough, most of the long-haired kids of the 1960s are the mothers and fathers of the 1980s, and they're scrambling to stay afloat just like everybody before them. They may use different slang words than I used when I was their age, and they may not bat an eye at attitudes and practices that could have sent a person to jail in my time, but they are still the same, and they want pretty much the same things people have always wanted. A place of safety for themselves and their children, a little food, a little warmth, and some one other person with whom to share their lives. Because in the long run when all of life's battles are just about over that's all life boils down to, the essentials. We all work

45

like hell for the luxuries, and if we are very lucky we end up with the necessities.

I think that's why with a mind filled with memories like an overcrowded attic, I can look at my life and say that the two most important things in it are my work and my wife, Alexandra.

I'm not insulting children or grandchildren. They're important, of course, but in a secondary way because they have their own lives. We all love each other—the Camutis are a close family —but not in the same way that Alex and I do. We not only love each other, we need each other. We are each the center of the other's life. And we should be. I've known Alex since I was nine years old.

I won't say Alex shaped my whole life—the proud Camuti heritage and my years in the military life had their effects—but she certainly put up with it, and I know her constant love and patience with me has made me a better person than I would have been without her.

I've heard enough people in my time describe me as feisty, a bantam rooster, a curmudgeon and a little Napoleon to concede that maybe there's something in all those names and words. But I know this: Alex has stayed with me as my wife for sixty years as of April 1980 so I can't be too bad.

That "proud Camuti heritage" I mentioned refers to the fact that I can trace my family's history all the way back to the 1700s and a long, unbroken line of physicians in Parma, Italy. Camutis headed the medical school there and one of them earned and passed on the hereditary title of Count to succeeding generations. There was even a Camuti who served as physician to the Duchess of Parma who was the daughter of the King of Spain. Technically speaking, if I was still in Italy and things were the way they were back then I would be Count Louis Joseph Camuti. What I am instead is a count of no account, which is okay by me.

It was my grandfather, a fabric merchant, who first broke the Camuti medical tradition. Though his son, Gaspare, my father, went to medical school, he left when my grandfather died and went into the fabric business to support the family.

46

I was born in 1893 and named Louis Joseph. The brother who followed me was Joseph Louis. When I was nine, my father booked first-class passage aboard the *La Gascogne* and moved the family to America and our first home in the New World on MacDougal Street in Greenwich Village.

I'll never forget my first day in America. It was March 17, 1902, St. Patrick's day, which may explain why I came home from a look around the neighborhood with two black eyes, a gift from the neighborhood toughs. Perhaps the local street gang didn't think it right for a kid to be speaking Italian—the only language I knew—on St. Patrick's Day. Or maybe it was the Buster Brown outfit I was wearing that set them off. I couldn't understand one word they said to me before the fists started flying.

For our first weeks in Greenwich Village, my brother and I were outcasts huddling together. I think what set us apart and made us tempting targets was a combination of the way we dressed, the way we spoke, and the fact that we were proud Italians who spoke proper Italian, not a dialect. And then one day everything changed.

We were walking in Washington Square Park, keeping eyes peeled in every direction for sudden attacks when suddenly, up ahead, we saw two children with their mother, and they were dressed the way we were. We ran up to introduce ourselves, shaking with excitement, and laughing for the first time in weeks. At last, we weren't alone.

I didn't know it at the time, but the pretty little girl, Alexandra Landi, would one day be my wife.

Her family was a prestigious one. Her father was Fidardo Landi, the sculptor. His father-in-law, Alessandro Biggi, was not only a sculptor of note but also the Dean of the School of Sculpture in Carrara and the Mayor of Carrara.

The Landis and Camutis embraced each other and a lifelong friendship began. Not only did everyone like everyone else, everyone needed everyone else. We had found people we could speak with in this confusing new country where even the Italians spoke English or a dialect that was difficult for us.

The friendship stayed strong even when my father moved us up to Leland Avenue in the Upper Bronx, where I began my schooling at P. S. 36. From that school I went to Stuyvesant High School, then the only technical high school in the city school system, and a two-hour trip each way to and from 14th Street in Manhattan. While my family takes pride in its ancestry, I was most proud that I had come to this country not speaking a word of English and by graduation time was invited to be a charter member of the Stuyvesant High School branch of Arista, the high school honor society.

If my language changed during those high school years, so did I. I can't say I grew to be six feet tall or even close to it, but I changed from a boy to almost a man. With that change came the change in my feelings toward Alexandra Landi. Somewhere along the way Alex ceased being a friend, became my secret crush, and then the girl I knew I would one day marry.

During those same growing-up years, my father had become a successful wholesaler of Italian products, which meant he could afford to send me to college. Because gasoline engines were just coming into use for farm machinery, and because I spoke a pure Italian—thanks to Sunday grammar lessons from my father—I saw myself living high in Italy as the representative of a large farm-machinery company based in Auburn, New York, that had expressed interest in me shortly after I entered Cornell. Along with my required courses, I took electives in agriculture, and dreamed of Alex and me in Italy living as man and wife in a villa that looked across a vista of grape arbors and smiling faces.

The dream exploded in 1914 when the company told me that America would be shipping cannons, not farm machinery, to Europe for a long time to come. I turned to medicine, the centuries-long practice of Camuti men, and I flipped a coin: heads, veterinary medicine; tails, human medicine. The coin landed heads up. The next year at Cornell, I began doubling up in my work, combining the agricultural studies that I was already involved in with the first year of veterinary school.

Alex and I became engaged during my junior year at Cornell. To be nearer to her, I transferred to New York University at Bellevue to complete my veterinary studies, and I got a part-time internship with a veterinarian named Miller.

In the way that all people in love want to do something magnificent to prove to the one they love that they are indeed worth loving, I showed off to Alex as a veterinarian. I spayed her gray Persian kitten, Suzette. I don't mean that I put Suzette under the knife just to show off. Suzette was at the age when she should have been spayed, so who could possibly do it better than young Dr. Camuti? Of course, I had never spayed a cat before, but I had certainly studied how to. Big shot that I was, I didn't even ask Dr. Miller to supervise. Looking back, all I can say is that Suzette's surgery was the longest, toughest operation I have ever performed. Happily, both Suzette and I survived it, and good sport that she was, Suzette never held it against me.

When it began to look definite that America would soon be entering World War I, I wanted to enlist. I felt I owed it to the country that had taken my family in and had allowed us to grow and prosper. But when I tried to join up, I was told that I was a medical student and therefore exempt.

What I most wanted to be in was the veterinary corps, but with only incomplete studies to offer I knew it was hopeless. But I did have two years of ROTC at Cornell behind me. That had to be good for something. In 1916, I decided to try for the cavalry.

A professor of mine introduced me to a veterinarian, Dr. George Goubeaud, who was attached to Troop C of the First New York Cavalry located near Ebbet's Field in Brooklyn. Dr. Goubeaud took me to see Major McClear, who liked me and arranged for me to take a physical.

The cavalry rule at the time was that you had to weigh two pounds for every inch of height. At 5 feet 6½ inches and 125 pounds I was shy 7½ pounds. I was near tears. Luckily, the examining doctor took pity on me. He said, "I'm going to do something unorthodox. I am going to leave this room and shut

49

the door behind me. You'll notice that there is a drinking fountain in this room."

The minute the door closed behind the doctor, I ran for the fountain and began to drink. I gulped water until I thought I was going to drown internally. But when the doctor returned and put me on the scale again I was within a pound and a half of the weight minimum. He passed me.

The trip back to my parents' home in the Bronx was a nightmare. I practically sloshed my way to the subway, and I had to get off the train at almost every stop to find a men's room. I kept praying that the train wouldn't come to a halt between stations. If it did I was sure to be a public disgrace.

At the end of 1916, I entered the National Guard and found myself spending my evenings patrolling the aqueduct at Elmsford, New York, to protect it from possible German bombing attempts. On evenings that I wasn't at Elmsford, I was training with other recruits in Brooklyn. Large parts of every night were spent in long commutes back to the Bronx, where I would try to focus my tired eyes on my schoolwork.

It wasn't long before the dean at New York University at Bellevue called me into his office. He had learned how I was spending my evenings—"It's impossible," he said—and told me that my grades had dropped so badly that I would have to repeat the school year. I didn't see how repeating a year would make me any less tired for my studies, so I decided to drop school until after the war.

I had barely learned to stay on a horse when word came from France that additional horses were not needed over there. The cavalry became horseless.

The year was 1917, and I was a first sergeant at the Remount Station at Camp Wadsworth, Spartanburg, South Carolina. It was an area of corrals packed with horses that were no longer wanted by the artillery and the cavalry. Obviously, I was not located in a hot spot of wartime activity.

If life at Remount seemed dull, it soon turned into a nightmare when a contagious disease, shipping fever, showed up among the horses. The order came down to destroy the sick animals. I didn't expect that to be my job. After all, there were veterinarians all over the place. But when I learned how army horses were destroyed at that time, I could see why the buck was passed down to the sergeant level.

It was a messy and nasty job. Horses were shot, and too often a bullet would ricochet or miss its mark, and the animal suffered. If I was going to do the job, I decided that there had to be a better, surer way, one that would be painless to the animals.

I had the soldiers who worked with me build parallel fences —just wide enough for a horse to walk between—with a platform at one end on which I could stand. I stationed myself there with a hypodermic syringe filled with ten grains of strychnine which I would inject directly into the animal's jugular vein. The horse would topple to a swift and painless death. The only pain in the whole procedure was mine at having to kill such beautiful and trusting animals.

I told myself over and over again that the animal was sick and could not be saved. Wasn't I really sparing it pain? Yes, but it was something I had to remind myself of every day. I knew that bringing the peace of death to an animal was as much a part of being a veterinarian as helping a dog to give birth to its puppies, but still I suffered. I guess I was still a kid, and like all kids who think of becoming doctors, the first thought is of life. It is only later on that you have to face death as part of the job.

When I was discharged with the rank of second lieutenant in January of 1919, a flu epidemic had struck my camp veterinary hospital. Over a hundred men died. I don't know how I came to be released—maybe I kept quiet when I felt the early symptoms —but I arrived home with a fever of 103.

I guess I was too feverish to think straight, or too much in love to bother to think at all. All I knew was that I had been away from my fiancée for too long to be stopped by a mere 103 fever. When did a fever ever stop a second lieutenant?

I just dropped my duffle in my room and headed straight out the door in my uniform. One minute I was perspiring, the next shivering, but I kept heading downtown to the office where Alexandra worked. Luckily, I had the good sense not to kiss her. The romance was on again.

In time the fever passed, but not the one I felt every time I looked at Alexandra Landi. The "cosmic urge," as I call it, didn't subside at all.

I wanted to get married right away. Five years of being engaged to, but never alone with, the woman I loved was much too long. Why should we wait any longer? I had no doubt that I could support a wife. Hadn't I risen through the ranks to second lieutenant? That must say something good about me. I could type with two fingers and I had experience in administrative work. It seemed obvious to me that any smart company would snap up this returning veteran for an important job right away.

I talked things over with my father, who immediately set me straight. He pointed out that a bachelor's degree in agriculture wouldn't take me very far in New York City. "And I think you can forget what you learned in the service. My advice to you is to finish veterinary training. If you don't want to practice after graduation, you can try some other line of work, but you will always have veterinary medicine to fall back on."

What he said made sense, and I knew it, even as I tried to argue with him to see things my way. And when I mentioned the cosmic urge, he smiled and said he knew a sure cure. Cold showers. "Do what I say, Louis. Finish your studies and then get married. I'll send you to Europe for a years's honeymoon. And when you come home, there will be five thousand dollars waiting to get you started."

I took cold showers and went back to Bellevue.

After what seemed like a lifetime, but was only January of 1920, I was graduated from the New York University School of Veterinary Medicine. Alex became my wife on April 6, 1920.

Considering how long we had waited to be together as man and wife, what happened after the wedding makes no sense to either one of us today. But there must have been a reason back then.

Instead of going straight from our reception to the room we had reserved at the Hotel Pennsylvania, Dr. and Mrs. Camuti went to the circus at the old Madison Square Garden at 26th Street and Madison Avenue.

When we finally got to our hotel room, the cosmic urge still did not get satisfied. We spent most of the night like a couple of dopes picking up the rice that fell from our clothes and luggage because we didn't want anyone at the hotel to think we were newlyweds!

The next morning, we went to the boat that was to take us to Europe for our year's honeymoon. At last, we were alone with no telltale rice on the floor, no one to disturb us. And the moment the ship pulled out to sea, Alex became seasick and stayed that way across the entire Atlantic. I took more cold showers. If the Guiness Book of Records wants us for "The Bride Who Remained a Virgin for Two Weeks in Constant Company of Her Consort Who'd Been Waiting for The Big Moment For Almost Six Years," they can have us. It must be a record.

Needless to say, things changed when we left the ship. In Italy, we made Alexandra's grandparents' house in Carrara our home base while we toured Italy and fell deeper in love. In Venice, where we spent a month, the honeymoon came to an end sooner than expected. We learned that Alex was expecting our first child.

We booked passage home so that our baby could be born in the United States of America. Nina, the first of our two children, arrived on March 4, 1921, the day that Warren Gameliel Harding was inaugurated as President of the United States. We were living in the Bronx home of Alexandra's mother. I was a proud father, but I was also a scared husband, the head of a family to support, and the world was not beating down my door.

Chapter 5

WHILE I CAN'T REMEMBER how my first client ever found me—I was in the Bronx and she was in Brooklyn—I remember everything else about the case. And if the lady is still alive, I'll bet she remembers me, too.

It was a weekday morning and I was looking through the newspaper, trying to figure out this new world we were entering now that the war was over.

Everything was changing in postwar America, and the changes affected everything, even the practice of animal medicine. Horses had once been the bulk of any veterinarian's practice—and certainly, they constituted the bulk of my experience—but now, suddenly, they were a disappearing breed. The newly popular automobile was removing them from the streets of the city. The carriage horse, fire horses, wagon horses, trolley horses—they were all going. Veterinarians who once looked down their noses at treating household pets were now more than interested in treating them. My problem, of course, was not one of switching from the treatment of horses to cats and dogs, but of finding any patients.

And then the telephone rang. The lady's voice was warm and sad. "Dr. Camuti, can you come to Brooklyn? My dog, Tiny, has to be put to sleep."

I didn't even stop to ask what the matter was with the dog. I said I was on my way.

I had just enough money for carfare both ways and to buy a bottle of chloroform at the neighborhood pharmacy. It wasn't until I was seated in the subway train that I began to wonder about what was wrong with Tiny—I pictured a small dog about the size of a cocker spaniel—to warrant his being put away.

Today, of course, I would refuse to accept such a request until I had checked the animal out thoroughly and was convinced that it couldn't be saved. But then I was young and desperate to prove to myself and the world that I was indeed a veterinarian. And you had to have at least one client for that—this one was mine.

It took almost two hours to get to the address I had been given, an apartment on the third floor of a brownstone. The woman who opened the door was middle-aged, a thin lady with a worried face. Behind her, I could hear a dog barking very healthily.

Tiny turned out to be a St. Bernard who seemed surprisingly frisky. I was startled by the animal's size and by its seeming state of good health. But I assumed it was a sick dog or the woman wouldn't have wanted it put to sleep. Back then, I automatically believed that everyone was in his or her right mind, and that people who had pets loved them.

Today I know better. As I said, "All of my clients are normal, but some are more normal than others."

I told the woman to bring her dog into the bathroom. I followed her in. She said, "I know you'll understand, but I just can't be in the apartment while you do it, Doctor. I'm going out for a walk. I'll come back after."

I nodded, and she left, closing the door behind her. I sat down on the closed toilet and fished the bottle of chloroform out of my jacket pocket. I took a towel off the bar by the sink and began to open the bottle. That was when I made my big mistake—I didn't realize that the bathroom was so small and that there was no ventilation. But between my own nervousness at what I was about to do and trying not to look at Tiny, who was licking at my hand, I don't think I knew where I was.

The last thing I remember was pouring chloroform into the towel.

I came to on the floor of the bathroom staring up at the ceiling. Tiny was licking my face, and the woman was glaring down at me.

I pulled myself to my feet. I had to hold onto the sink because the room seemed to be swaying and my knees felt as if they had turned to Jello. The woman opened her mouth to say something, but I cut her off. "No charge," I said, and lurched from the apartment.

It wasn't a great start at being a veterinarian.

My first real office was in New Rochelle. Somehow, I heard that they had lost their city veterinarian, and I went up to see the authorities, applied for and got the job. I opened my office on the second floor of a building on Main Street, right next to the police station, and began to wait for patients. I was certain it would be a very short wait. After all, New Rochelle was a wealthy community.

The high point of what turned out to be a brief stay in New Rochelle was one that still sends chills through me whenever I think of it. There was a rabies epidemic in town, and one morning the police called me to say that they had a homeless dog tied up in the station house that they thought was rabid. They were going to shoot it and they wanted me there to check the brains afterwards for rabies.

When I arrived, the dog was downstairs tied to a post. I had to take only one look to know the animal was rabid. I was standing beside two police officers with drawn revolvers. For some reason, the dog just kept glaring up at me, making low snarling sounds. Then the first officer fired at the dog. His bullet missed the animal but severed the rope. The dog lunged straight for me. I thought I was a goner for sure, but at the last second the other officer dropped the rabid animal with his shot.

I left New Rochelle shortly afterward. It wasn't because of

the rabid dog, but because the postwar boom was over, and the citizens of New Rochelle, like people all over, found themselves financially strapped. Too often I would treat a patient, only to be told by the client to "charge it." I didn't need that. I figured if I was going to starve, I might as well do it in New York City.

My next office was on the second floor of a building at West 10th Street and Greenwich Avenue in Greenwich Village, where Alex's cousin had a wholesale coffee business on the ground floor. Most of the telephone calls I got in this new office were from Alexandra asking if the phone was ringing. I told her it rang every time she called me. I spent the rest of my time trying to figure out why every sick cat and dog in Greenwich Village recovered the minute I moved into the neighborhood.

Luckily, I wasn't completely dependent on the animals of Greenwich Village for my livelihood. I was taken on as a veterinary inspector by the New York City Health Department. The work, which took only about five hours a day and brought in $1,700 a year, involved everything from checking out reports of dog bites to inspecting slaughterhouses and food-processing establishments.

Between working for the city, trying to build a practice in Greenwich Village, and commuting to the Bronx, I found myself pretty busy, though not very rich. But I felt I was getting somewhere. As time went by, the office telephone rang more and more, so I figured satisfied clients had to be talking about me. And in December of 1923 I passed out cigars to announce the birth of my son, Louis, Jr. The Camuti family was complete.

Suddenly it was 1929, and the world crashed. The night it all ended, I sat up late in the living room staring out of the window at the Grand Concourse. Alex and the children were asleep. I just sat there watching automobiles go by, wondering what if anything was ahead for me.

Finally, Alex came out and told me that I was accomplishing nothing sitting in the dark and feeling sorry for myself. "We'll manage," she said. "We always have."

57

I took her hand. That was my Alex. Always on my side, always believing in me.

"Well, look at it this way," she said. "You can stay up all night and worry, or you can get a night's sleep and worry in the morning when you're rested."

Alex had always had a way of putting things in order for me.

Very soon afterward, a friend sent me to see Grace Agramonte, head of the Humane Society in Mount Vernon, New York. She confirmed what I had heard, that Mount Vernon could use another veterinarian. She recommended the vacant clapboard house at 16 East Broad Street, next to her own home, as an ideal site for a veterinary hospital. She also helped me locate a house on Harding Parkway for my family.

The four Camutis, my mother-in-law, and the Camuti pets, Suzette and Fluffy moved in. We'd either make it or go bust in Mount Vernon, that's all there was to it. In the back of my mind, I wondered if Mount Vernon was going to be another New Rochelle for me, but I tried not to show my fears to Alex or the children. If Alex was worried, she never let me know.

I didn't know it right away, but Mount Vernon was the beginning of my life as a veterinarian. I don't mean that I started my house-call practice for cats then and there. That didn't come until later. For many years I conducted my practice, both in Mount Vernon, and later in offices on Park Avenue as other veterinarians did, seeing my patients in my offices.

It was that, working day in and day out with all kinds of animals, I discovered myself and my purpose for being alive. I'm not saying that I think I was put on this earth to be a veterinarian. Maybe I was and maybe I wasn't—I don't know. I don't go in much for that kind of thinking. What I mean is that I realized that I was truly happy and satisfied doing veterinary work, healing animals.

Maybe being an animal doctor would never bring me half the wealth I had once dreamed of placing at Alex's feet, but that didn't seem to matter anymore. And I know it never mattered to Alex. I was happy and she was happy, and that was enough.

Chapter 6

It surprises me when I look through my card files how many names mean nothing to me today, especially when my notations tell me there was a long string of office visits or house calls. Yet I can come across another card that has only one notation, and I remember the person vividly.

I suppose that time has a way of sorting people out, storing some in the memory, discarding others. The ones I remember most clearly are the special people. Some are special to me because of long, close associations or a kindness they performed. Others are special because they fall into the category I describe as "more normal than others." In other words, the oddballs.

If this book is about me, then it must also be about the people who have made an impression—good or bad—on me. One way or another (and not always because of a cat patient) these characters are important to me.

Reuben Crispell is a good example. He was a highly successful lawyer whose dog, Franzl, I took care of, but Franzl isn't the reason I remember Reuben Crispell. He stays in my mind because of a license plate.

Franzl, not the license plate, brought us together. The Crispells lived in Bronxville, and since Mr. Crispell's work often kept him away from home, he used to send Franzl, an Airedale, to me during the summer months while the family was in Vermont. I must have asked, but I don't remember the answer, why Franzl didn't go to Vermont with the family. I do know that I didn't mind having Franzl with us for the summer.

How Franzl felt, I am not too certain.

One summer morning I got a call from Reuben Crispell, who was at his Bronxville home, about a mile away. He sounded fairly testy. "Camuti, where's Franzl?"

"What do you mean? He's over in my hospital right now. In fact, I think this is the morning George is going to give him a bath. Why?"

Crispell exploded. "Because I'm standing here shaving, and I'm looking out the bathroom window. I can see Franzl swimming in the pool!"

I checked with George Mosby, my right-hand man. Sure enough, Franzl had escaped from him in the middle of his bath and leaped out of the ground-floor window. George was relieved to know where the dog was. "I guess Franzl's washing off the soap," George said.

Luckily, Reuben Crispell didn't hold Franzl's escape against me or I wouldn't have gotten the license plate I had wanted.

For whatever crazy reason that has always attracted me to gags and gag gifts, I had always wanted license plates to commemorate my veterinary medical practice, and I don't mean the standard DVM kind. Reuben Crispell, through some special pull he had up in Albany, got me the plates I coveted: VD 1.

Alex wasn't thrilled when I put the plates on my car, but I was. I liked seeing the startled look on people's faces when I pulled into a curb, or watching in my rearview mirror for the moment when the driver behind me spotted the plates.

At first it amused me when kids would shout to one another, "Don't touch that car or you'll catch it," or when policemen would laugh as they wrote out the parking tickets I was always collecting. But after awhile the joke wore thin. I think the breaking point came one night as I was waiting for the light to change at Park Avenue and 33rd Street. Two marines—I think they were drunk—started cracking jokes at the top of their voices while a crowd gathered to see what it was all about and I sat waiting for what seemed like the longest light in the world to change. The last thing I heard as I put the car in gear was, "The son of a bitch brags about it!"

That did it. A joke's a joke, but I realized I was making a fool of myself wherever I went. I had my plates changed to the more standard DVM.

Not that I have them today. In time, another yen started working on me. Thanks to friends and clients like Phyllis Levy, I got the license plates I had wanted for over fifteen years. They were presented to me at a mammoth party on October 5, 1976. I was amazed that all these people who didn't know each other —Alex had helped supply names and addresses!—had gotten together just to honor me.

The license plates were the greatest present I have ever received. And it took a telephone call from the former mayor of New York City, John V. Lindsay, to his friend, the Commissioner of Motor Vehicles up in Albany, to swing it. From that day to the day I stop driving, if you ever see a car with the license plate CAT you'll know the man behind the wheel is me.

Doris Bryant had come to New York City from somewhere out West, and she was most helpful to me in developing my cats-only practice. Doris was devoted to all cats, but Siamese were her specialty. She bred them.

Doris was always very pale. Her skin had the look of alabaster to it. She seemed like a delicate statue come to life. In fact, she resembled—at least, to me—the large ceramic Siamese cat that stood in her pet-supply shop window.

But there was nothing of the cold statue about Doris Bryant. She was a warm, outgoing person and a bit of a character. In her shop on West 11th Street in Greenwich Village she sold all sorts of cat accessories—scratching posts, litter pans, carriers, toys—everything a cat owner could want. Cat lovers came to her from all over the city, and she usually was very helpful to a customer. But if someone came in that she didn't take to, Doris had no hesitation about throwing him out. "That's not for you," she'd say, or more bluntly, "You don't like cats well enough, get out!"

Our twenty-year friendship began when I got a call to her shop to treat one of her cats. From that first visit on, Doris decided I was the doctor for her. She put me in charge of all her cats, and whenever someone came into her shop who needed the services of a veterinarian, Doris recommended me.

This was all back in the mid-1930s when there were no special medicines for cats. Everything back then was for dogs. With Doris's encouragement I began developing a line of medications for cats, and Doris stocked them in her shop. She even sold them through the mails, a practice that stopped with the Food and Drug Act of 1938.

Doris would place ads in pet journals for the medications: Medicine 1, for vomiting; Medicine 2, for something else, and so forth. I didn't make any money from these medications, but that didn't matter to me. I was a doctor, not a pharmacist. I was interested in the medicines in terms of sick cats who might be far from veterinary help. I was also interested in helping Doris to stay in business through the Depression years. My deal with Doris was that she was to pay me for the cost of the medicines and the containers. The small profits she made were all hers.

Doris was married to a man named Mack who was a vice president with a large New York advertising agency before he lost his job early in the Depression. But Mack was a resourceful man. To make a living he baked little pastry cups and filled them with hamburger. He took them around and sold them to the speakeasies while Prohibition was still on, and then to barrooms all over the city. Between his pastries and her shop, they managed.

There were thousands of incidents in the twenty years I knew Doris Bryant, but there is one that stands out as typical of her. To me, it shows Doris's whole attitude toward life. She got on with it. Her troubles were her own to handle, and she didn't bother other people with them. When her problem was settled, then—and only then—you might find out that Doris had been through something.

The time I'm thinking of was when I received a letter from her telling me what cat medications she needed more of. At first, the letter seemed no different from dozens I had received from her. In fact, I didn't discover the difference until I went to work to prepare the medications. The letter read:

> Dear Dr. Camuti,
>   We need more medications. Please send me:
> 1 dozen Number 3
> 2 dozen Number 1
> 1 dozen Number 5
> I divorced Mack
> 1 dozen Number 2.
>
> Doris.

Of all the clients I've seen over the years who are "more normal than others," I think I'd give the top honors to a beautifully groomed, soft-spoken gray-haired lady whom I'll call Mrs. Jones.

All veterinarians are used to men and women showing up in the waiting room in various stages of distress over what their pet is going through, or what they think their pet is going through. But when George Mosby came into my office at 65 Park Avenue and said there was a lady with a sick dog in the waiting room, I could tell by looking at his face that this was something special. George looked as if he had been hit with a brick.

I told him that the woman would have to wait her turn. George shook his head and said he thought I ought to see her quickly because her dog looked strange to him.

Trusting his judgment, I finished the animal I was treating at the moment and signaled to George to bring the woman in.

Mrs. Jones made such an impression of breeding and taste that I had to take her seriously as she held out her pug dog to me. It was made of papier-mâché!

"What can I do for you?" I asked.

"My dog is full of ticks," she said.

I looked at her. She was serious and concerned. I realized that Mrs. Jones was getting senile. "How long has he had them?" I asked.

"Well, they are all over the house now, and he's scratching himself to death."

"May I have a look?"

She handed the pug to me. I could see that the tail served as a handle by which you could lift off the rear end. The pug had been made to hold candy.

I turned the dog every which way, pretending to study it. Then I said, "I can only find one tick on him."

Out of the corner of my eye, I could see George looking from me to the papier-mâché dog to Mrs. Jones. I could imagine what he was thinking.

"I'll tell you what we'll do," I said. "I'm going to give you some powder, and once a day you sprinkle some on your dog's tail. It should keep the ticks off."

At first I had thought to give her some mineral oil as a salve, but I realized it would soak into the papier mâché and probably the tail would crumble. I didn't know what that would do to Mrs. Jones. So I got down a container of unscented talcum powder and poured some into a box and handed that to her.

About a week later, George came running into my office. "She's back!" I knew exactly whom he meant.

"I don't think that medicine is doing him much good," she said, and she seemed rather annoyed with my lack of medical knowledge. "And it seems to be making him nervous. I put him on the window sill and as soon as the hotel flag starts to wave in the wind he barks and barks for me to move him away."

I tried to soothe her. "Well, they do get nervous sometimes."

"And another thing. The hotel maids don't want to come and clean in my apartment because of the ticks."

"Tell you what. Use the medication for one more week, and then we'll try some other treatment."

She agreed, and asked, "What do I owe you?" She took out a thick roll of bills.

I was happy that she had come to me instead of some unscrupulous person who could have fleeced her outrageously. "Today, you don't owe me anything. When we finish the treatment I'll discuss the fee with you."

A few days later she was back again. It was one of those afternoons when I had a full waiting room. Instead of sitting and waiting her turn, Mrs. Jones stood in the middle of the room. When George came into the room, she announced, "I want to have my dog put to sleep."

There was nervous shifting about over the room as people looked at the papier-mâché dog.

"The doctor will see you shortly," George said. "Please have a seat."

The next time he returned, George noted that several people had left. He brought Mrs. Jones and her pug in to me.

She repeated her request. "Okay," I said, "you just leave him here and I'll take care of everything."

I thought I had seen the last of Mrs. Jones. When she left my office, I put the toy pug on a shelf in my office as a remembrance of her.

Several weeks went by, and then there she was again. She spotted George as she entered the waiting room. "Do you remember my dog? You put him to sleep three weeks ago. Well, I want him back."

There was a man with a cat carrier seated in the waiting room. He took a quick look at Mrs. Jones, grabbed his hat and the cat carrier and left. He never came back.

George came into the examining room and told me what had happened. I took the candy-box pug from the shelf and put it on my treatment table. I told George to bring in Mrs. Jones.

She was delighted to see her pug, and scooped it up into her arms. "Has he been eating well and did he enjoy his stay?"

I assured her he was fine. "And his tick problem is completely cured, too."

This time she insisted on paying me. "I couldn't think of it," I said. "He was such good company, I should pay you."

That was the last time I ever saw Mrs. Jones. I heard through some friends at her hotel that her brother had moved her to his house in Massachusetts.

George was happy that she had moved away. Whenever he spoke of her, he always said, "We lost more clients because of her."

But I missed Mrs. Jones. For her sake, I hoped that there was a good veterinarian nearby in case the ticks came back.

Just mentioning George Mosby as a part of other people's stories is not enough. George was too important in my life for a passing reference.

George Mosby was both my assistant and my friend, though I doubt that George would have thought of himself that way. George referred to himself as my "man" and that was all there was to it. There was an invisible line between us, one of George's own construction, and he lived on one side of that line and I on the other. If I had had a rough day at the New York office and wanted to stop for a cup of coffee before driving home, George refused to go into the restaurant or diner with me. He didn't regard that as proper, and he would sit in the car and wait.

I don't suppose many of today's Blacks would approve of George, but that wouldn't bother him. He didn't want to associate with them. "We were gentlemen down South," he would often say. "These are all roughnecks."

George had been born on a plantation in Staunton, Virginia, where his parents had been slaves. He had no birth certificate so he never knew for certain how old he was. While he was still a child, his family moved North and he spent most of his life on the south side of Mount Vernon.

My guess is that George was about forty years old when Grace Agramonte, the lady who had helped me to establish myself in Mount Vernon, brought him to me. He was six feet tall and very thin, a divorced man with two grown children. He told me that he was an orderly at a nearby hospital, but he wanted to change jobs. I think it was that Southern-gentlemanly way of his, as well as his hospital experience, that made me decide on hiring George almost immediately. I never had cause to regret the decision.

The coming of George changed a lot of things around my Mount Vernon animal hospital. Before George, I only had an occasional animal overnight, but with George on the premises day and night I could take in more patients. That was how the problem with Inky started.

Inky was a black cat who belonged to one of the women in a U. S. senator's office. He came to me when the lady's mother became ill and the daughter found herself spending her lunch hours and evenings at the hospital. She told me that she didn't have time to give Inky the attention and affection he deserved. I offered to take the cat as a boarder at my hospital until her mother recovered. The lady accepted my offer.

Inky seemed to adjust to life at our hospital very quickly. After a few days, I decided to allow Inky the run of the place when there were no other patients around. Either George or I would pop Inky into his cage during office hours.

Inky was a friendly fellow, warm and outgoing with his affections to George and myself. In almost no time at all, he fell into the habit of greeting me at the hospital front door each morning with a purr and a tuck of the head as he rubbed himself against my trouser leg. And then one morning, he wasn't there.

George and I checked through the whole hospital. No Inky. For several days we continued to look for Inky, but we never found a trace of him. Finally I gave up and confessed to Inky's mistress that he had disappeared. She took it pretty well.

As time passed and business increased at the hospital, Inky gradually drifted from my mind. Then one morning I arrived at the hospital to find George sitting on the stoop. He was shaking his head and mumbling to himself.

"The noises again, George?" I said, referring to the noises George often mentioned coming from somewhere near his attic bed. I never paid too much attention to George's talk of noises since he could never describe them or pin them down in any way. I dismissed the sounds as George's imagination combined with something like air in a radiator pipe or a window rattling.

George nodded. "The noises, and Inky."

He told me that after he had gone to bed the noises had gotten so bad that he had gotten out of bed determined to find the cause once and for all. He found some gaps between the flooring of his room and the ceiling below. He put his hand into the widest of the spaces, reached down and felt something furry. He grabbed hold and pulled. He felt the fur coming free of whatever it was attached to. Up came the pelt of a black cat. It was Inky. The cat had obviously gotten up into the attic, been trapped under the floorboards and died of starvation without ever making a sound when we had gone through the hospital calling his name.

The skinning of Inky left George shaken, but not out of superstition. In fact, he told me that down South where he had come from black cats were considered lucky.

George continued sleeping up in the attic, and according to him the noises continued. He never discovered the cause.

Though I never called him on it, I always knew that George was practicing veterinary medicine among the poor people in the Black section of town. It didn't bother me at all. In fact, it pleased me, and it made me feel warm about George that he cared enough to want to help people who couldn't afford to bring their animals to a veterinarian.

Too often, at the end of a day, when the last client had left the office, George would begin a casual discussion with me about someone he knew whose cat or dog wasn't "acting right." I'd ask what he meant by that and George would describe the symptoms for me in detail. Then I'd tell him what the complaint sounded like, and I'd give him a small bottle of antibiotics or a tube of ointment.

I never asked George what he did with the medications I gave him, and he never volunteered to tell me. But we both knew the other knew what was going on. George was taking care of his patients just as I was caring for mine.

Only once in all our years together did we ever have trouble. In the small washroom off my operating room I always kept a bar of Cashmere Bouquet soap for washing up between patients. One day I noticed that there was a fresh cake of soap on the sink. That struck me as odd since I distinctly remembered putting out a fresh cake the day before. At first, I thought it was just George being meticulous about things around my surgery. But when I discovered that there was a brand-new, unused bar of soap on the sink three and four times a week, I became suspicious. Could George be stealing it? It seemed impossible.

Finally I confronted him. "George, have you been taking the soap out of the sink?"

"Not me," George said. "I thought you were taking them home at night. When I come in in the morning and there's no soap, I open a new one."

"Why would I take the soap home when I want it here? We have soap at home."

"Well, don't look at me," George said. "It's not my brand."

Obviously, something was going on that George and I knew nothing about. But what was going on made no sense. Who would break into my hospital several times a week and steal only a cheap cake of soap?

We both started watching the soap as if it was made of solid gold. We spent the day periodically peering into the washroom to see if the soap was still there. It was. And it was there the next day and the day after that.

I noticed that the longer that cake of soap stayed in the bathroom, the less George and I talked to each other. Suspicion had set in between us. I know I began to silently blame George, and I believe he decided that for some crazy reason I was trying to frame him as a soap thief. It made a sort of cockeyed sense. With only two of us working in my hospital, the thief had to be one of us. And I knew it wasn't me, and George knew it wasn't him.

Then one morning as I arrived at the hospital there was George in the doorway grinning. "I know where your soap's been going," he said. "A rat took it."

"Oh?" I said.

George could tell I didn't believe him. "A big rat," he said. "I saw him dragging the soap right through a hole in the bathroom floor. I'll show you."

I got a flashlight and George showed me a hole where the floor joined the wall behind the toilet. I had never noticed it before.

I was still skeptical. I would not have thought that a place where cats and dogs were boarded, where clients and their pets came and went all day, was the type of place a rat would dare to show up. But rats were nervy creatures, and George had seen one with the soap. And there was that hole. I began to believe him.

George and I tried everything—except the obvious—to catch the rat. I bought traps of all sizes, some in which I think you could have caught a small bear. Nothing. I bought every type of cheese available, from the cheapest to the most expensive. Still nothing. In fact, we'd arrive mornings to find the cheese untouched and another cake of soap missing.

It was George who saw the solution. "If that rat likes Cashmere Bouquet so much, it seems to me we ought to try that for bait."

I set a brand new cake of Cashmere Bouquet deep inside the wire-cage trap, and the next morning, there he was. The rat weighed four pounds. His coat was as smooth and sleek as if he had been curried and cared for every day of his life.

"That's because of all your fancy soap," George said.

George was both an excellent assistant and the best dog groomer I have ever met. He worked very closely with me, even after 1945 when I closed down the Mount Vernon hospital and practiced only in New York City. With his hospital room gone,

70

George took an apartment in Mount Vernon and commuted daily with me to the New York office.

In 1947, George suffered a stroke that put him in a nursing home after he left the hospital. I visited him every evening after I completed my work in the city. I thought he was recovering, and we talked about the day when he'd be working with me again.

One afternoon, my son Louis called me at my office. He had just heard from George's daughter-in-law. George had died and was to be buried in Potter's Field.

I was furious. If neither of his two children nor the church to which he'd given so generously over the years would see that he got the proper funeral a man of his dignity deserved, then I'd see to it. George Mosby was not going into a pauper's grave.

I called the Kensico Cemetery in Valhalla, New York, where I have a family plot and purchased a single grave for George. He was buried as he had lived—quietly, properly, and with dignity.

As I will one day join George in that cemetery, I guess you can say we will be together again.

Chapter 7

I'VE HAD SEVERAL CLIENTS tell me that I am a saint because I make house calls for cats in New York City. "You have a true calling," another client told me. One even sent me a Christmas present with a card that read, "To the Albert Schweitzer of the cat world."

Well, that's fine for them, and I appreciate the kind thoughts, but frankly, I think of myself as some kind of nut. I know that if I were starting my practice today, I would never make house calls in New York City. The traffic, the parking—it's all impossible.

Truth to tell, I never planned the kind of practice I've ended up with. It just sort of happened while I wasn't paying attention. By the time I became aware of the changes in my practice and how it affected my life, I was too caught up in the new order of work to go back to anything so tame as sitting in an office waiting for patients to be brought to me.

World War II caused the change in me and the city. The war brought an influx of single people from out of town to the big city where jobs were plentiful. Older teenagers and recent college graduates broke away from their families to live in apartments. And at the end of the war, many of the returning veterans didn't go home to the small towns they had left at the beginning of the war.

It made for a city that had in it a lot of lonely people. In their search for companionship, they acquired pets, and in time, husbands and wives. And in the changing social standards that came in after World War II, it became normal for wives to work. The new breed of woman hadn't been raised to just stay home with the kiddies and run a house for her man. More and more, the only thing home during the day was the family pet.

Since most young couples couldn't afford domestic help—a scarce commodity in any case—more often than not I'd get a call asking if I could see Felix or Fido in the evening. Or if that didn't suit me, the next suggestion would be that if I would come to the apartment, the doorman would have the key for me.

Before I knew it, I was spending only about an hour a day in my office. The rest of the time I was running around the city with a large bundle of apartment keys. That didn't make great sense to me. I wanted my clients present so we could talk over their pets' problems or so I could explain how to use the medication I was leaving.

And so my hours changed. I'd start my house calls around four in the afternoon, work through the evening, sometimes as late as midnight, then go home and have supper with Alex, after which I'd do my bookkeeping, read a bit and go to bed around 4 A.M. to wake at noon and start the next day.

My breakfast is at one in the afternoon, lunch is around six or seven, dinner after midnight. Since Alex was living on the same crazy time schedule that I was, it wasn't long before she was joining me in my city rounds.

Granted I think Alex is the best company in the world—any person who doesn't feel that way about his mate has a marriage in a lot of trouble—but she serves more of a purpose on our rounds than just companionship. Alex is in charge of explaining to the police what we are doing parked in front of a fire hydrant.

Fire hydrants are the one sure parking space near any building so we head for them automatically. The problem is my nonmedical CAT license plates. When I had my VD, and later

VMD plates, there was a greater tendency on the part of the police to believe Alex's statement that her husband was inside making a house call for a sick cat. With CAT, they look rather skeptically at Alex, but she eventually convinces them. Or if they don't believe her, they decide that the dear gray-haired lady is a bit dotty and they leave her alone.

If Alex should ever lose her charm and her gift of gab I still have one more ace up my sleeve. I learned this one from Dr. Janet Briggs, who told me about the cat breeder who brought her Sacha and Dacca to her.

The breeder had sent his son to deliver the cats to Dr. Briggs while he waited outside. Dr. Briggs had a few questions about feeding her new cats and asked the youngster to send up his father.

As the breeder came through the front door of her building, the lobby-desk attendant asked the man if he wasn't concerned about leaving his car unattended and double parked. "They'll tow you away for sure, mister."

The breeder just laughed. "I never have to worry about that. I drive a hearse. Anyone who sees it thinks I'm inside picking up a stiff."

I've tucked that story away in the back of my mind for future use. Don't be surprised if some day there's a hearse driving around New York City with CAT license plates.

Anyway, that's how I've become a saint, and the Albert Schweitzer of cats. It just sneaked up on me. But try to tell that to a cat lover. For reasons I've never figured out, cat lovers are a fiercer breed than dog lovers, horse lovers, or anything-else lovers. It is these cat nuts who love their pets so fiercely that they divide the whole world into friends—people who like cats—and enemies—people who don't. These people invent and believe all sorts of nonsense about cats, from special foods that their cat must have to such bunkum as the idea that a cat will never overeat.

It is these same people that have spread the falsehood that cats are my only patients. Cats *are* my specialty, but can they really imagine that as a doctor I would refuse to see a sick animal because it wasn't a cat?

I used to say that if an animal will fit through an apartment door, someone in New York City will have one as a pet. In my time I have treated everything from honey bears to ocelots, though I have never understood why a seemingly levelheaded person would take into his home an animal that had the potential, when fully grown, to rip him apart. To the best of my knowledge, the clients who went in for "jungle warfare," as I refer to the raising of a jungle beast as a house pet, all survived their experience, (though they ended up poorer in pocket if their pet was the sort that required several pounds of meat each day). And most of them ended up heartbroken, too, when they had to find a zoo home for their would-be pet.

On a safer and saner level, I've come across some pets that were neither cats nor jungle beasts, but quite memorable in their own right. One of them was Anastasia, the pigeon that the Millers invited into their home. Anastasia was never my patient, but I'd meet him every time I went to the Miller apartment to tend to their cats.

Yes, Anastasia was a boy, only the Millers didn't find that out until after they had named him. The reason for the fancy name, they told me, was because they wanted the pigeon to know that he was something special. What made him so special to the Millers is that he was hatched on their windowsill. Anastasia's mother obviously didn't find her son as extraordinary as the Millers did because she promptly abandoned him.

I agreed with Anastasia's mother. He didn't look so special to me, either. Compared to the parrots, cockatoos, macaws and mynah birds that have crossed my path, Anastasia was just another New York run-of-the-park pigeon with slate-colored feathers and a faded rainbow of violet, green and purple bands around the neck.

But it wasn't looks that made Anastasia memorable. It was his personality. He was a highly social creature. The Millers' parakeet—which Anastasia ignored—wasn't half so charming. In fact, the parakeet had a habit of shooting his droppings at you if *he* felt ignored. That parakeet was a blue Annie Oakley. He would pick up his droppings from the bottom of the cage and fling them, with impeccable marksmanship, out between the bars at his target.

Anastasia was far above such vulgarity. His socializing began with sitting on Mr. Miller's shoulder or fluttering down on the dinner table, when the guests were seated, to walk around, cocking his head in pigeon fashion, as he scrutinized each guest. He never begged. Anastasia had too much dignity for that, but he could always count on at least one sucker in every dinner party slipping him a few crumbs.

Whenever I made a house call, Anastasia paid a flying visit to the table I was working on to look me over. I got rather fond of the little fellow, a fondness that promptly died when Anastasia learned his big trick.

It began one morning at the breakfast table—needless to say I wasn't there—when Mr. Miller dropped some toast crumbs on his shirt. "Come here, Anastasia," he called, and pointed to the crumbs.

The pigeon immediately flew over and picked the shirtfront clean. Then he got carried away with himself and poked his head inside Mr. Miller's shirt and began pecking at his navel.

Mr. Miller, who adored the bird, was thrilled. Anastasia loved navels! A new routine was born. Mr. Miller started putting crumbs and seeds in his navel for Anastasia. Every morning at the breakfast table, and every evening when Mr. Miller returned from his office, Anastasia flew in for a landing on his belt and poked his head inside the shirt to check him out for goodies.

Naturally Mr. Miller had to show me the great trick on my next visit. Anastasia performed on cue.

"Isn't that amazing?" Mr. Miller said, grinning with parental pride.

I thought it was repulsive, but I gave a safe answer. "He's certainly the only navel-picking pigeon I've ever seen."

Mr. Miller held out some seeds to me. "Go ahead, you try it."

76

I declined, but Mr. Miller wasn't put off until I snapped, "No pigeon has ever pecked at my navel, and I'm damned if I'm going to let one start now."

The Millers looked startled, and Anastasia cocked his head at me. "I'm sorry, Anastasia," I said. "Now, where's that cat I'm supposed to see!"

Then there were the monkeys, and New York is full of them. Naturally, I mean the kind with tails. While I can see the charm of a monkey, I frankly don't think they make such great pets. Lovable they may be, but they can also get pretty wild and messy. But as with any animal you can mention that someone has decided to make a pet, no matter how dangerous the creature or how repulsive its habits, when a would-be pet lover falls in love common sense goes out the window.

The Fitzpatricks, who were famous for those "Fitzpatrick TravelTalks" we used to see at the movies, loved and owned marmosets. Marmosets are tiny little monkeys that weigh only ten to fourteen ounces when full-grown.

The Fitzpatricks owned five marmosets—one male named Fritz, and his four wives. These South American jungle creatures lived in a special temperature-controlled room that had its own oil burner to keep the heat high year round. In the center of the high-ceilinged room there was a dried-out tree with branches for the animals to climb and jump around on. The walls had stacks of open shelves, another play area for the marmosets, who probably never had it so good back home.

I got a call from Mrs. Fitzpatrick when one of Fritz's wives was pregnant and seemed ready to deliver. As soon as I entered the monkey room I could tell which marmoset was my patient. Her abdomen was terribly extended. It was obvious to me that she was dangerously overdue. I decided to perform a caesarian on the little mother.

That I had come to help out one of his wives didn't impress Fritz one bit. If anything, he resented my intrusion into his domain. While I was discussing my plan with Mrs. Fitzpatrick

Fritz gave his wives the order and they jumped up onto the branch beside him, right over my head. Fritz screeched his next command, and he and his three wives promptly defecated on me. I was marmoset dirt from head to foot.

I had to go home and change. When I returned, Mrs. Fitzpatrick was on the telephone with a woman doctor at Polyclinic Hospital in New York who was studying the marmoset's ability to propagate in captivity. She, in turn, was relaying Mrs. Fitzpatrick's information to a doctor in England who was also studying marmosets. According to these two specialists, no marmoset had ever survived a caesarian section, nor even lived to get off the operating table. Obviously I was in a position to make medical history.

The operation was performed in the Fitzpatrick kitchen. As I feared, when I opened up the mother I found the baby dead and beginning to decompose. It weighed only an ounce less than its mother.

But the mother was alive—in weak condition, but alive. I carried her to a spare bedroom where I had an oxygen tent ready for her if she came through the surgery.

It broke my heart to look in at the tiny, almost human face staring sadly out at me. There was a tiny tear under each eye.

The strain of carrying her child for so long and the shock of the operation was just too much for the little creature. She lived only forty-eight hours.

That all previous records for marmoset survival had been broken meant little to me. I kept seeing that sad face that looked like a miniature of an elderly person. And those tears. I had failed.

Miss Petri's Luigi was a whole different package of monkey business. He was a capuchin, the kind of monkey that organ grinders used to take around with them.

Miss Petri spotted him in a pet-shop window, and Luigi's soulful expression dragged her right into the store. The owner of the shop recognized a softie the minute he saw one. He gave

Miss Petri a long, sad story about Luigi's being returned by its owner who was being transferred and had had to abandon the family pet. The homeless-waif approach hit Miss Petri deep in the heart, and suddenly she was the owner of a capuchin.

She took Luigi home and hung his cage in the kitchen over her dinette table. That way she could talk to him, and he could jabber back while she was working in the kitchen. Occasionally she would let him out, and Luigi would go swinging around the apartment by his prehensile tail. At night, Luigi slept in his cage tucked into a blanket made to his size by Miss Petri.

In no time at all, Miss Petri was completely taken with Luigi. She didn't know how she had ever lived without him, though she had to admit that if there was one thing about her capuchin she was not too wild about, it was his special diet. His usual lunch was worms that were imported from Japan, and his favorite treat was Mexican grasshoppers. He had two of those each day, one in the morning and one in the evening. Mexican grasshoppers, by the way, are the world's largest. They measure four inches across the wing tips.

A snack at other times of the day was usually fruit—apples, grapes, bananas. Occasionally he even took a bit of meat. But none of this human food could touch his favorites—worms and Mexican grasshoppers.

To give Luigi his due, I saw him eat a grasshopper on several occasions, and he had the table manners of a gentleman. He ate slowly and neatly, and never licked his fingers, though he did make lip-smacking noises.

After Luigi had been with her a few years, Miss Petri thought he might prefer the company of creatures more like himself. A friend referred her to an importer of wild animals, and through him she located and brought home two young monkeys.

Luigi went mad for them on sight and showered them with attention and devotion. When Miss Petri gave him a grasshopper or an apple he'd feed it to the other two, even though she'd made certain that there was more than enough food for all three. At night, Luigi wouldn't sleep. Instead, he covered his two charges with his blanket and sat up watching over them. I suggested to Miss Petri that she change Luigi's name to Luisa.

Miss Petri didn't think that was funny. She was worried about Luigi.

The lack of food and sleep finally weakened poor Luigi to the point where he could barely stand up. When I came to see him, I found a distraught Miss Petri and a capuchin that bore little resemblance to the once frisky Luigi. There was no doubt in my mind that the loving little monkey would die soon if something wasn't done quickly.

The next day, Miss Petri took the two new monkeys back to the place where she had gotten them, explained the situation and left them there.

Luigi was grief-stricken for a few days, but then he began to eat and sleep again. Within a short time he was his old frisky self, swinging around the apartment.

Peace reigned again in the Petri household, or it did until Miss Petri met Mr. Winters. Though she was in her forties and he was in his early fifties, neither of them had been married before. But suddenly they found each other and discovered that they had a great deal in common. Both taught in colleges, both enjoyed going to concerts, and both were rabid fans of the New York Yankees.

Friendship quickly turned to love for Miss Petri, and she hoped to marry Mr. Winters. It should have been a happy time for her, and it was, except for Luigi, who obviously detested Mr. Winters from the start.

The more Luigi saw of Mr. Winters, the more he disliked the man. It didn't help matters that Luigi was kept locked in his cage when Mr. Winters was expected. Whenever Mr. Winters arrived, he was greeted by a barrage of angry monkey chatter, a vicious monkey face with teeth bared, and the sound of the cage bars being shaken with rage. If Mr. Winters tried to make peace with all the sweet talk he could muster, Luigi drowned him out with screeching.

Once Mr. Winters tried bribery. He brought Luigi a bag of

peanuts which he held up to the bars of the cage. Luigi looked at the bag and Mr. Winters suspiciously. Finally he accepted the bag. Mr. Winters thought he had made some progress, and Miss Petri was thrilled. Then, from his cage, Luigi emptied the bag and flung the peanuts as far as he could throughout the room.

At last there seemed to be a change. One evening when Mr. Winters arrived at Miss Petri's apartment Luigi actually stayed calm. The usual thundering rampage didn't take place. Instead, Luigi just sat in his cage, holding onto the bars, peering quizzically out at Mr. Winters.

Thrilled with this sudden thaw, the couple decided to let Luigi out of his cage. The monkey went through his usual leaps through the apartment and ended with a swing atop a bookcase.

Thinking this evening marked the breakthrough that could save his hopes for a wedding, Mr. Winters asked his fiancée for something to feed Luigi. Miss Petri went to the kitchen and came back with a piece of banana.

Mr. Winters took it and sat on the arm of the couch. He held up the banana for Luigi to see, and began coaxing the animal in a soft, cooing voice. "Here, Luigi, look what I've got for you. Luigi, nice monkey, smartest, cleverest, prettiest monkey . . ."

Luigi came down from the bookcase with his usual loose, bouncy gait and went toward Mr. Winters' outstretched hand.

Miss Petri was thrilled.

Luigi took the piece of banana, then sank his teeth into Mr. Winter's finger.

Mr. Winters told me what happened. "Luigi not only bit my finger, but he wouldn't let go. My fiancée was screaming, 'Don't hurt him! Don't hurt him!' and she meant I shouldn't hurt Luigi, not that Luigi shouldn't hurt me. Meanwhile, its teeth are still in my finger, and the little monster is wrapped around my arm. Its nails had scratched through my shirt, and my arm was bleeding as much as my finger. I'm yelling for her to toss some water on Luigi, to call the police, to call you, to do *something,* and she's only worried I'll hurt him. She wouldn't toss water on him because he might catch cold, and she refused to call you, the zoo or anyone. Suddenly, I decided to stop trying to shake him off. I just rapped him on the nose and he let go."

Miss Petri was so shocked and furious that Mr. Winters had hit Luigi that she refused to accompany him to the hospital emergency room where seventeen stitches were taken in his hand and arm.

Mr. Winters left the hospital in a deep depression. He knew he'd survive the suturing, but he wasn't certain that he could survive too many further attacks by Luigi. He didn't look forward to a life without Miss Petri, but Miss Petri came with Luigi. That damned monkey was all that was keeping them apart!

Miss Petri must have done some thinking, too, because she telephoned Mr. Winters the next day to apologize for sending him to the hospital alone. They arranged to see each other that evening.

Once again, Luigi was silent when Mr. Winters arrived. Miss Petri let the monkey out of his cage, and as usual, Luigi went swinging around the apartment. Only this time Mr. Winters kept both his jacket and gloves on. He ignored the monkey completely, and didn't even turn his head to look when Miss Petri said Luigi was smiling at him from the top of the bookcase.

A few minutes later, Luigi leaped onto Mr. Winters' shoulder. He ducked instinctively, certain the monkey was going to bite a chunk out of his ear. But instead, Luigi wrapped his arms around Mr. Winters' neck and snuggled his head next to Mr. Winters'. Miss Petri began to cry for joy.

It was the rap on the nose that Mr. Winters had given Luigi that had turned the tide. The pecking order had been established. Miss Petri became Mrs. Winters shortly afterward. Man, wife and monkey lived happily ever after.

While I don't take on new clients with dogs, I certainly wouldn't turn one away with an animal that was suffering. And in my time I have had many dogs for patients. In fact, I treated many cats and dogs belonging to Episcopalian ministers. The reason for that was Bishop Horace Donaghan. Though I'd given up my dog practice years before we met, I thought it would be unchristian to turn down his request that I take care of his new pup. After all, Bishop Donaghan was the Bishop of the Diocese of New York.

The Bishop had been born in England, kept a summer home in Surrey, and was quite a good friend of the Queen Mother. The royal family raises corgis, and they presented the Bishop with a male pup. He named it Monarch in their honor.

When he brought Monarch home to his residence at St. John the Divine in New York City, he asked me to come and check the pup over. I was surprised, considering the puppy's royal background, to discover that it had a tapeworm and only one testicle. I suggested that the Bishop send Monarch back to the Queen. "Or at least ask her to look around for the missing testicle."

To put it mildly, Monarch didn't like visitors. In fact, he bit people. Whenever the Bishop conducted a meeting or gave a party, Monarch was locked up. Nevertheless, one day I was called to the residence because Monarch had bitten a Con Edison meter reader.

According to New York law, when a doctor treats a case of dog bite it must be reported to the Health Department to make certain that the dog isn't rabid. The Bishop had sent for me to attest to Monarch's health, which was easy enough for me to do. But I still had to see the dog for eight days to fulfill the Health Department's requirement.

When I showed up the day after the biting incident, I thought there was a riot in progress behind the residence. People were lined up all along the fence and I could hear Monarch barking for all he was worth and two men shouting. One of the shouting men was standing outside the gate waving a piece of paper.

Inside the yard was the Bishop's Philippine houseboy trying to catch Monarch and shouting at the man outside the gate. The man with the paper had come to serve the Bishop with a summons because of the biting incident. Monarch had decided that the man looked just as bitable as the meter reader, and the houseboy thought the man had come to take Monarch away. It was a scene of total confusion, and I enjoyed watching it for several minutes.

Then I went over to the man and told him I would take the summons inside. He thought I was crazy to imagine I could get inside the gate without getting bit. But I knew that Monarch was afraid of me. Whenever I showed up it meant a shot or some sort of poking around that the corgi didn't like, so he usually ran.

Which is exactly what happened when Monarch heard me talking to the man with the summons. The dog took one look in my direction, stopped barking, put his tail between his legs and ran for his life. The entire crowd along the fence looked at me as if I were the devil himself. I pretended not to notice as I opened the gate and walked right in.

I can't say why, but shortly after this incident Monarch calmed down. He didn't have any more run-ins with meter readers or process servers. In fact, he became quite likable and lived to a ripe and peaceful old age.

Of all the dogs belonging to Episcopalian ministers I've ever tended to, my favorite was Gretchen, a dachshund, who lived with Father Leslie Lang at St. Peter's Church, Westchester Square, in the North Bronx.

Granted, I have always been a pushover for dachsies, but Gretchen was a charmer. Father Lang was very proud of her enormous ears, her golden-orange coloring and shiny black tail. It made her look as special as he thought she was.

When she was only a few weeks old, she accompanied Father Lang on a trip to Nassau. Since the idea of his beloved Gretchen traveling anywhere except at his side was unthinkable to him, Father Lang gave Gretchen half a sleeping pill before boarding. She spent the entire flight nestled against his neck at the top of the airplane seat.

Because he had a great deal of traveling ahead of him, Father

Lang left Gretchen in Nassau for a few months with Father Thomas Lee Brown at St. Barnabas Church. Father Brown, on leave from St. Peter's in Westchester for a tour of duty in Nassau, had bought Gretchen for Father Lang and so was considered a suitable dog sitter. Though she regularly accompanied Father Brown to services and once routed a burglar from the clergy house kitchen, what Gretchen is most remembered for is marching in the Bay Street parade for the Patronal Feast of Saint Matthew's. Gretchen came down the center of Bay Street in a low-slung strut that focused every eye on her, and she knew it and loved it. Gretchen was definitely a people dog. If she was left alone, she would howl so loudly that guests at the nearby Royal Victoria Hotel would hear her and complain.

A few years after she returned to Father Lang's rectory, three new dachsies—Roger, Heidi and Wie Gehts (German for "How goes it?")—joined Gretchen, who quickly taught them who was the "mother superior" in that household.

Suddenly, when Gretchen was eight or nine years old, her hind parts became paralyzed. I was called immediately. It was my first meeting with Gretchen, and I fell in love with her within seconds. And I knew it was mutual because whenever I came to the rectory after that, Gretchen, who managed to pull herself around the house on her two front legs, would drag herself over to greet me.

Father Lang hung a silver medal of St. Roche and his dog on Gretchen's collar. The Bahamian houseboy sent a shilling home to Nassau for his family to have blessed by their obeah man in hope of a cure. And I visited Gretchen every day for a month to give her alternate shots of cortisone and B_1.

After each day's shots, I'd set Gretchen on her back on the kitchen workbench for her daily massage. All of Gretchen's lower bodily functions had to be stimulated by hand. The dachshund either understood that the massage helped her or she liked it. All I had to do was call out, "Where's my girl?" and Gretchen would come to me, dragging her back end, waiting for me to pick her up and carry her to the kitchen.

It was either the shots, the massages, St. Roche or the obeah man's blessed shilling—or all of them combined—but on the thirty-second day, Gretchen stood up on all four legs, shook herself straight and walked. Father Lang, the Bahamian house-boy and I stood with tears running down our faces as Gretchen wagged her long-still tail to show us what great shape she was in.

A few years later Gretchen developed a breast tumor. I performed the surgery to remove it in St. Peter's rectory kitchen. Gretchen, who was as strong as she was lovable, came through with flying colors.

Shortly after her surgery, Father Lang was assigned to another parish. Though it broke his heart to leave the dogs behind, Father Lang decided that Gretchen was getting too old to be asked to make an adjustment to new surroundings, and he didn't want to separate the dogs, who were quite devoted to each other. So he left them at St. Peter's in the care of Father Brown, who had returned from Nassau.

The next excitement at the rectory was caused by Heidi's pregnancy. Heidi was due to deliver just when Father Brown had to be away. He left the church and the expectant mother in charge of Father Hayes, who called me the minute Heidi began her labor.

I rushed right over and was pleased when Father Hayes offered to assist me. We moved Heidi from her box to the kitchen table which Father Hayes had covered with newspaper. "No good," I said. "Take that stuff off and get some clean old towels, and cover them with an old blanket you don't care about."

I talked softly, assuring Heidi that I would do everything I could for her as soon as the table was ready. I know many people put down paper when kittens or puppies are expected, but I don't approve. The stuff may be disposable, but the animals sometime shred and eat the paper, and it's not good for them.

When her delivery table was ready, I placed Heidi on it. Heidi was a wonderful patient and helped me every step of the way.

She even stayed flat on her back, instead of on her side which most animals favor.

When the pup burst out, Father Hayes, my volunteer assistant, gave a frightening moan and passed out. I watched him sink to the kitchen floor like a punctured balloon. I left him there. Heidi needed me more than he did.

I lifted out the puppy, severed the umbilical cord, removed the placenta, and gave the tiny newborn a gentle rub with a towel to clean him up and get his circulation going. Heidi, meanwhile, had jumped off the table, curled up in her bed and waited for me to bring her son to her.

It had long been decided that if Heidi gave birth to a male its name would be Peter since it had been born at St. Peter's. Peter it was.

With mother and child settled in for the night, I turned to Father Hayes and helped him to his feet. He looked sheepish. "Some assistant," he muttered.

The years slipped by, and one night I got a call from Father Brown. Gretchen had grown old gracefully, and now her time had come. She was dying. I knew there was nothing I could do, but out of love for Gretchen I went to the rectory. I was met at the door by Father Lang, whom Father Brown had telephoned. The tears running openly down Father Lang's face told me that Gretchen was already gone.

He told me about it. When he arrived, Gretchen was lying on the floor. When she saw Father Lang, she crawled over to him, too weak to stand. She tried to get into his lap.

Father Lang picked her up and carried her to her basket bed. For the second time in her life, he gave Gretchen half a sleeping tablet. He sat down beside the basket so that she could see him. While he whispered private words to her so that Gretchen would know she was not alone, she closed her eyes and went to her maker.

Chapter 8

As FAR AS I am concerned there are two kinds of cats: city cats, and others. Oh, I know that a cat's close relatives are lions and tigers, strictly outdoor types, predators capable of taking care of themselves. Therefore the very idea of there being such a thing as a city cat, one who lives its entire life indoors, sounds unnatural. Well, fine and good, but it doesn't cut much ice with me.

I think city cats are terrific. Show me a lion or tiger that can adapt itself to any size apartment and never miss the outdoors, which city cats do all the time. And there are some lucky cats who have both city and country homes and adjust quite easily to two different life styles, especially if they have been going from one home to the other since kittenhood.

There are two reasons why cat owners take their pets to the country with them. The first is that they love their pets and hate to leave them behind. The second is that a cat has a high old time when it gets outdoors and can run around.

But I know this as a fact, and it's one every cat owner ought to consider: The cat that spends his life indoors lives the longest. Those cats that spend part of their lives indoors and part outdoors have shorter lives. And those cats who live all of the time out of doors—even if they come home to eat and to visit—have the shortest lives.

The reasons why an indoor cat lives the longest are obvious:

the indoor cat never runs the risk of being run over by a car, or of catching diseases from other cats, or of suffering injury in animal fights. Its owner can protect it from toxic plants, parasites and poisons. That's why I see so many old cats in my city practice, more than I'd see if I had a country clientele. Most of my clients take my advice and keep their cats inside—not that many of them have a choice, since they are apartment dwellers.

As for country kittens that are brought to the city, they adapt as easily as if they had been born in Times Square. Litter-box training, about which some people have trepidations, doesn't bother cats at all—not even a cat who has always done his duty out of doors. Just show a cat his box as soon as he enters his new home and starts sniffing around, or carry the cat over to the litter box once or twice right after it has fed and sit it down in the litter. The cat will get the idea.

Balaban and Eartha Katz, the Frankels' black litter mates, were born in the country and raised by their mother until they were almost three months old, at which point the Frankels got them, and the two brothers became city cats on weekdays and country cats on the weekends. They had no trouble adjusting to their city-country life. The only thing it took the boys a few weeks to learn was that when they were in the country they didn't have to come running indoors to the litter box when nature called.

One of my clients, who had a rodent problem in his West Side Manhattan leather-handbag factory, decided to "hire" some cats from his summer place near Lake George. He brought back a mother cat and her three kittens, all of whom had been abandoned on his country property. He quickly discovered that his new family were terrific mousers and didn't seem to miss the mountains at all. So far he's employed three generations of that family at his factory.

Visiting his cats was one of my few chances to see a mother cat training her young in the fine art of hunting. The mother, a gray female with white and black stripes, would catch a mouse and bring it live to her kittens. If a kitten didn't catch the mouse when she let it go in front of him, she would cuff him on the nose and bring the mouse back for him to try again. After each of her kittens had learned to catch the mouse, she would show them how to kill it and eat it.

Once in a while I have had clients tell me about a mouse that got into their apartment—or their country house—and that their city-bred cat didn't do anything about it. Joe Fleming, a large gray city cat who spends his summers in the country with Tom and Alice Fleming, both writers, is an example. The Flemings once trapped a mouse in a downstairs closet of their summer house. Tom picked up Joe and tossed him into the closet with the mouse. After an hour of total silence from the closet, Tom opened the door. The mouse ran out of the closet, shot through the parlor and out onto the front porch where it worked its way to freedom under the screen door. Joe Fleming calmly sauntered out of the closet and went about whatever he was up to before the Flemings interrupted him.

Why didn't Joe do what every cat is supposed to do? It could be that Joe wasn't interested in the sport of mousing, or because his mother never had the opportunity to teach Joe before he went to live with the Flemings. It could also be that Joe, who once had a weight problem before he slimmed down, just wasn't hungry.

Some city cats—not Joe Fleming obviously—love the hunt so much that they are forever killing things, like neatly wrapped Christmas packages, stray bits of string, and Cellophane from cigarette packages. In her fascinating book *The Cat,* Muriel Beadle says the rustling of Cellophane mimics the sound of mice in an underground burrow. Never having heard a mouse in a burrow I can't swear to that, but her theory would explain the almost universal appeal of Cellophane to cats. Whatever the reason, I wish people wouldn't toss crumpled Cellophane to their cats. Cellophane can be dangerous if swallowed.

People in the country often complain that they have to run a "chop check" before they let their cats into the house. It's one thing for your cat to rid your garden of moles, but you don't want them alive and squealing in your living room. Ditto rabbits, frogs, snakes, chipmunks and birds. I know it is a very popular belief that a cat brings its catch to its owner because it wants praise. Well, not according to Muriel Beadle. She says that the cat is trying to train its owner, just as its mother trained it.

It is generally believed that a cat that gets lost in the country or the city can survive longer than a dog in the same situation. Certainly dogs are more dependent on their owners for food. Though the matter is still being debated by those who study it, I suspect there is truth in the cat's ability to survive longer on its own. Even after generations of apartment living, and a mother who may not have taught it what to do, a cat could probably survive for a while outdoors. Some atavistic hunting traits would probably surface.

Too often a window is left open and a cat wanders away. Assuming the cat isn't killed in traffic, it probably won't starve as long as it has its claws to help it catch its dinner.

Even as I write this I can feel my blood starting to boil. Anyone who declaws a cat is indulging in a cruel and barbaric practice. I've always been against it, and nothing can change my mind.

People who have cats declawed usually do so for one of two reasons: to prevent being scratched by an aggressive cat or to preserve their furniture. Such people are obviously thinking only of themselves, not of the pets they are supposed to love. For their own selfish reasons they put their cats through a surgical procedure which is severe, both physically and emotionally.

Emotionally, the trauma may last a long time, and in some cases forever. Very often a cat is declawed without any attempt on the part of the owner to train the animal first to use a scratching post. The cat never had a chance. In fact, I've known of cases where a prospective owner demands a cat be declawed before he'll adopt it. I certainly would never give a cat to such a person because the request itself is an indication that the household is not suitable to a cat.

Moreover, it also upsets his balance. Contrary to popular belief, the cat does not have a perfect sense of balance, any more than it has nine lives. If cats were born with an innate sense of balance, how come so many of them fall out of windows and off terraces? And if they have nine lives, how come so many of them don't survive the first fall?

As far as I am concerned, clipping a cat's nails, providing him with a scratching post and training him to use it are the answers —never declawing.

A cat uses his scratching post to keep his nails in readiness. Since the claws grow, just as our nails do, the cat uses the post to keep his claws at a proper length. Sometimes if there is nothing on which to scratch, and the nails become too long, a cat may bite them off.

An owner who loves his cat will clip its nails regularly, because if the nails grow too long they can turn under and penetrate its delicate pads. This can cause a painful infection. The proper way to clip a cat's nails is only along the white, curling edge, never down to the pink part, which is colored by blood.

Few cats like to be given a manicure, but if you can hold your cat's paw while he is snoozing, you can usually snip a few nails before he's awake enough to give you a rough time. Another good time to try is just after the cat has eaten and is feeling logy. Of course, you may turn out to be lucky and discover that you have one of those rare cats that doesn't mind the procedure at all.

The big trick is to train your cat to use his scratching post in place of your rugs, furniture or draperies. As to which scratching post to get for your cat, I'd recommend sisal as the best. It is sturdy and it has a different texture from the things in your home that you cherish. If you get your cat a carpet-covered scratching post—and there are an awful lot of them on the market—you only confuse the cat. Why is carpet on his scratching post okay, when carpet on the floor is not?

No one is fool enough to tell you that a scratching post will add to the decor of your home. But it is a necessity, and it doesn't take up much room. Any place your cat frequents regularly—near the food bowl or the litter box—will do. Phyllis Levy, who has a top editorial post with a leading magazine, lives in a very smart East Side apartment in New York City. Her living room is done in beige. So is the scratching post and the ceiling-high retreat on which her Barnaby and Tulip like to perch.

My favorite scratching-post story belongs to Mrs. Kahn. Mrs. Kahn kept her cat's scratching post in the dining room. It just ended up there because the cat never used it no matter where it was placed. It stood in its corner year after year, ignored by everyone except one of Mrs. Kahn's housekeepers. Evidently the woman had studied it for a long time without a clue as to what it was. Finally, when the woman was leaving Mrs. Kahn's employ, she got up the courage to ask about "that thing" in the dining room. "I've always wanted to know, but I didn't want to seem rude," she began. "Does it have something to do with your religion?"

What do you do when your cat heads for your sofa instead of the scratching post? You say, "No!" firmly and lift the cat up and carry him over to the scratching post. Make scratching motions with his paws and say, "Good kitty, good kitty." The lesson may not take right away, but in time he should catch on.

Most cats like to have a good scratch following a nap, so watch for those moments. You could move the post near to his favorite sleeping spot so he'll see it as soon as he awakens. But whether your cat gets the idea of using the scratching post or not, and even if he claws your expensive sofa to ribbons, I am still opposed to declawing.

While we're at it, I'm also against cosmetic changes for dogs such as trimming the ears and docking the tails.

Some people accuse me of practicing a double standard. Since I'm against altering nature when it comes to cats' claws and dogs' ears and tails, why do I alter cats? Because there's no connection. The life style of a domestic cat has changed so much from that of the cat in the wild that neutering is essential.

In order for the cat to propagate, nature has given it periods of sexual urge which vary both in intensity and in frequency. In the female these periods cause a great deal of anguish and frustration, resulting in a state of nervousness manifested by outcries that prove her discomfort. The female often refuses food, and these periods of sexual heat keep those who stay constantly in season too thin.

People who say that a spayed female becomes obese and lazy miss the whole point. When you spay a cat, you remove the reason for its emaciation, thus allowing nature to bring the cat to its normal weight.

As to the male cat living under apartment conditions, his life would be one of frustration if he were not neutered. The unneutered male often turns on its owner with no provocation and may inflict serious injury. Furthermore, the smell of the unneutered male's spray on the furniture is enough to drive the most devoted cat owner from the apartment. Once the spray is in your furniture, nothing can remove it. What a cat sprays is urine, but the odor of an unaltered tom's urine—even in a litter box—is much stronger than that of his neutered brother's.

Females, by the way, can and occasionally do spray. The reasons for a cat's spraying are many and varied. I've known some cats who would spray to punish an owner because they resent something he has done—or not done. A tom may spray to establish his territory or to alert other cats to his presence. Granted this reason would seem invalid for a single cat that is always housebound, but not if you realize that it is an involuntary reversion to the outdoor way of life. Even if your cat sprays after he's been altered, the odor is not so bad.

One would assume that a cat who is the only pet in a city apartment and who never goes outside is free from danger. Unfortunately, there are windows and cats love them.

Cats love to bask in the warm sunlight on the windowsill and watch the world go by. Fine and good, but never assume that your cat is so happy at home or so afraid of the outdoors that he wouldn't go out through an open window. Cats can squeeze themselves through unbelievably small window openings. Any cat owner who claims to love his pet should install a sturdy, full window screen before he considers opening the window even a fraction.

Cats should never be allowed on open terraces. They are curious creatures and will walk to adjoining terraces and disappear, or worse, fall off.

Cats do indeed fall and hurt themselves. Granted, cats can fall and right themselves, but not always.

I've known cats that have fallen ten or fifteen feet and broken their legs. But then again, I also remember a telephone call a few years ago from a client who told me her cat had fallen thirteen stories. She had left the window open while she was doing her spring cleaning.

"Why are you calling me?" I asked. "Call the ASPCA, and they'll come for the body."

"You don't understand, Dr. Camuti. He fell, but the doorman says he is trying to climb back up the brick wall!"

"I'll be right over."

I couldn't believe it. But sure enough, when I got to the lady's apartment, there was her cat. He was a little shaky, but he was fine, except for one tooth that had been knocked out.

Another good reason for having window screens in an apartment, aside from keeping cats in, is that they also keep cats out.

Elizabeth and Michael Charrier, who live in the Murray Hill area of Manhattan, always left their fire-escape windows open in good weather. The windows were fully barred and they didn't own a cat, or at least not a permanent cat. Elizabeth often fed homeless waifs who seemed to know the Charriers were hospitable to cats. Word must have gotten around the back alleys of the neighborhood because there was a daily parade of four-footed visitors who came for a handout before pushing on.

All the cats, with the exception of one, would sit patiently outside the Charrier window waiting for Elizabeth to come with the food bowl. The exception was a tough old tom with one chewed-up ear who often showed up early in the morning before the Charriers were awake. If he found the window down, the tom would beat against the pane to wake them. If the window was open but there was no food waiting, he would howl until Elizabeth came running.

It had to happen, of course. One day, a black-and-white tom decided it was silly to fend for himself when the Charriers seemed so hospitable. He stepped through the bars, picked out a comfortable chair and waited for Elizabeth and Michael to discover him and feed him. The Charriers named him Bogart.

It was obvious on examination that Bogart was not a street cat. He had been neutered. Possibly he had gotten an attack of wanderlust, or perhaps he had been mistreated at his former home. There was no way of telling how long Bogart had lived the street life, but there was no doubt that he much preferred living with the Charriers. Though they still continue to leave the fire-escape windows open, Bogart never goes out.

The Charriers were lucky with their open-window policy. Charlotte Abbott wasn't.

Miss Abbott owned a pretty female tabby, Maroushka, who had the run of the first-floor townhouse apartment and the garden. In good weather Maroushka loved to step out into the garden, nibble a few blades of grass, then curl up on the flagstone patio for a nap.

But one day a male Russian Blue appeared from somewhere in the neighborhood. Almost daily he came bounding over the fence to chase Maroushka out of her own garden. He even followed her right into the apartment, and once he caught Maroushka in the middle of Miss Abbott's living room and severely mauled the tabby.

Miss Abbott was furious, but there was nothing she could do but keep her windows shut. That didn't strike her as fair, since the Russian Blue still came around to stalk Miss Abbott's yard, while poor Maroushka had to stay indoors.

One day, while speaking with Belle Livingston, a neighbor, Miss Abbott mentioned the Russian Blue. Miss Livingston told her that she, too, although catless, was also bothered by the "mobster cat," as she called him. He had come in through her open bathroom window and stalked through her entire apartment. "But it only happened once," Miss Livingston said. "That mobster saw this little stuffed figure of a wolf cub—it's only about a foot high—that I have, and it scared the daylights out of him. He went shooting out of my apartment. Since then, I've kept the figure on my windowsill, and I haven't seen that dreadful cat since."

Miss Livingston loaned the wolf-cub figure to Miss Abbott, who placed it at the garden entrance to her apartment. The Russian Blue came around the next day, took one look at the cub and leaped over the fence and away. After only a few days, he stopped coming around, and Maroushka was able to enjoy her old life again.

George Freedley, who died in 1967, was theater critic for the *Morning Telegraph,* curator of the theater collection at the New York Public Library and secretary of the New York Drama Critics Circle. Cats were as much a part of George's life as the theater was. Through the years I looked after the health of Mr. Cat, Princess Amber, Master Sable and Mr. Moonlight for George. Mr. Cat was the most remarkable of the lot, and George recorded his antics in a 1960 book entitled, appropriately, *Mr. Cat.*

In all the time that George and Mr. Cat shared their lives together, George never had screens on any of his windows, and Mr. Cat, a notorious wanderer, would always return. He was the original cat burglar.

Mr. Cat would come and go through the bedroom window, which led onto the fire escape of George's third-floor apartment at 19 East 55th Street. The assortment of terraces and fire escapes on that block made it possible for Mr. Cat to cover a great deal of territory. And he often came back with a souvenir of his travels—a glove, a hat, even a toupee. George never knew where Mr. Cat went, so he could never return the loot. Though George claimed to be embarrassed by Mr. Cat's thieving, he did keep everything he was presented with in a box that he would trot out to show to guests with some pride.

Just in case you are beginning to find Mr. Cat charming—and if you get hold of George's book in which he describes Mr. Cat in loving terms—I'd like to say that I thought Mr. Cat one of the meanest critters I ever met. Mr. Cat hated me, of course, and I wasn't too wild about him.

When George had to bring Mr. Cat to see me at my hospital, he told me that the animal growled all the way up and all the way back in the taxi. To be fair, he probably hated the confinement of a carrier as much as he hated me. Mr. Cat was in such a state by the time he arrived at my hospital that often George just lifted the top of the carrier and I gave the cat his shot without taking him out of the box.

If ever I needed proof that cats should be treated at home instead of at the veterinarian's office, Mr. Cat was it. Not that Mr. Cat liked me any better on home territory. When I gave up my last office and started exclusively making house calls, I found that Mr. Cat hated me just as much on his own turf. And George couldn't hope to shut Mr. Cat in the bathroom in advance of my visits as other clients do. Mr. Cat would have slipped out as I slipped in. So even at home, Mr. Cat had to be put in his carrier before I arrived, which didn't improve our relationship at all.

As a thief, Mr. Cat seemed to go through phases of collecting in his work. For a time he seemed to be fascinated with tape measures and brought home a large assortment of them. George assumed that he probably lifted them from the workrooms of the women's hat and dress shops that backed onto George's block. Many of Mr. Cat's prettiest trinkets such as bits of fabric, ribbons and pieces of lace seemed to come from these shops. Then, one night, Mr. Cat brought home a woman's straw hat. George was very upset, but what could he do? All the shops had burglar alarms and bars on their windows, but obviously Mr. Cat slipped right through. And George couldn't see himself walking from shop to shop with the straw hat asking if it was theirs, and then telling the owner that his cat had stolen it. George was certain he'd be sent to an asylum.

George decided to do nothing. To thank him, Mr. Cat topped himself and brought home a nearly finished gray skirt. George found it hard to believe that in as congested a city as New York no one had noticed a cat with a skirt in his mouth.

One evening, just after George had returned from a theatrical opening, Mr. Cat appeared with a gray suede glove. He dropped it proudly at George's feet with his usual *mmrrph,* and waited for a response. George had long given up on shaking a finger at the animal and saying "Bad cat." It had had no effect on the thief. George merely shook his head wearily, picked up the glove and put it on his dresser.

A few nights later, George was telling a guest in his home about Mr. Cat's thievery. He brought out the gray suede glove and showed how well it fit. "If only he'd bring me the other one," he said, just to make conversation. Then he returned the glove to his dresser and brought out the box of Mr. Cat's loot to show the visitor, not noticing that Mr. Cat had slipped out the window.

About an hour later, Mr. Cat appeared with a gray suede glove. At first, George assumed that Mr. Cat had picked up the glove from the dresser, but when he went to put it back he realized that the cat had brought home the mate. There was nothing to do but have the gloves cleaned and wear them, which he did for years.

Lillian Gish, who was a friend of George's, found it difficult to believe that everything in the booty box had been brought home by Mr. Cat. "You know, George," she said, "I really can't accept this. I think you've just given him all these things to play with."

Mr. Cat who was sitting nearby, stood up and left the room. He slipped out through the bedroom window and returned shortly afterward with a black velvet bow, which he dropped at Miss Gish's feet. George insisted she take it as a gift from Mr. Cat.

Years later, I met Lillian Gish at the memorial service for George Freedley. We'd both been asked to speak. She spoke of his love for the theater, another friend spoke about George's library work, and I spoke about his passion for cats. It was a meaningful service and I believe George would have been pleased. The things he loved had been spoken of.

My only regret is that I forgot to notice if Lillian Gish was wearing the black velvet bow Mr. Cat had given her.

Chapter 9

LET ME MAKE IT CLEAR about me and my pedigree. Earlier in this book, I mentioned the "proud Camuti heritage," and that I come from a long line of Italian counts. I also said that I am a count of no account. I mention all this again because I am about to talk about cats and pedigrees, and I suppose a lot of people are going to get upset about how I feel about pedigrees.

I am proud of my family, who they are and who they were. But that's it. It doesn't make my family any better than anybody else's. I should hope that everybody takes pride in his or her own family tree, even if you come from a long line of fish peddlers.

Pedigrees burn me up. They have nothing to do with the way you love a cat or how the cat loves you back. And if there is anything more important than love in the relationship between a pet and its owner, I don't know what it is.

Frankly, when someone tells me, "My cat has a pedigree a mile long," I mentally shake my head in pity. *Everyone* has a list of ancestors a mile long whether they know who they were or not. Unless you are going to breed a cat for money the parentage doesn't mean a thing. Some of the nicest cats I know are common domestics, also known as alley cats.

The whole business of pedigrees is pushed by the pet-shop owners so they can jack up the prices on cats. It's beyond me why anyone would spend hundreds of dollars on a kitten from a pet shop when every ASPCA, animal welfare league and half the cat owners in the world have kittens they will gladly give away free to good homes. The reason has to be tied up with ego or the need for a status symbol or some other such nonsense.

Obviously I don't think much of this showing off, but I can understand it to some degree in the case of a fancy breed of dog. At least, the dog gets walked outdoors where someone can see it with its master and say, "There's Mr. So-and-So with his dog. He must really be doing well to have a dog like that." But who, aside from friends and family, gets to see who owns the supercat that cost a fortune, since cats don't have to be taken out and walked?

I'm happy that what dogs have gone through for the sake of the human ego hasn't happened with such frequency to cats. With dogs that have become fashionable—the wirehaired fox terrier, the cocker spaniel, the poodle—the breeders have gone to work to improve the bloodlines. And what happens? They may get purity of breed, but they kill off whatever personality traits made the animal popular in the first place.

Boxers are a good example of what I mean. The old boxer was a much more likable dog than the ones you see today. But when popularity struck the breed, there were just so many available, and everybody and his sister wanted the new prestige dog. So the breeders went to work to meet the demand. They started breeding the animals too closely within the same family, and as a result, the new boxers are highstrung and can be vicious.

In cattle, the desire was for bigger udders for more milk. So they bred and bred the Holsteins, and what they got were cows that are more susceptible to diseases such as tuberculosis.

Some human geniuses and some handsome animals have resulted from inbreeding, but by and large it's a pretty risky business—with people and with animals.

I've never been closely associated with a breeder or a cat store, and I won't be. That would be working both sides of the street, and it goes against my grain. I've made it my policy to cut myself off from the producer and the seller in order to protect the purchaser. I think it's the best way to keep oneself working for the best interest of the cat and the owner.

One pet shop in Manhattan that sells fancy cats lets their clients have a new kitten examined by a veterinarian before plunking down the couple of hundred dollars purchase price, only there's a hitch in the deal. They stipulate, "Any veterinarian but Camuti." They know how zealous I am about checking out a kitten and telling people to take it back if it isn't healthy. If the kitten has a fever, runny eyes, a limp or a skin condition, it should be returned. And especially if it has a respiratory disease. This may be chronic and can spread to other cats in a household.

Let's face it—if you are going to get a kitten from a pet shop or a breeder you are running the risk of getting a sick animal. You're better off taking a kitten from a family whose cat had a litter and where you know the state of the mother cat's health. Second best is buying a just-weaned kitten from a shop or breeder that guarantees the kitten's health. It's not that shop owners and breeders don't care about their animals—many of them do—but they are dealing with large numbers of cats all the time. The chances of infection spreading through the entire cat population at their places have to be great.

Breeders also take chances. When they breed a cat for show purposes they are risking the cat's health every time they show it. They are continuously bringing their show cat in contact with other cats, and they are letting the cat be handled by men and women who have just handled other cats. Has anyone ever seen a pet-show judge wash his or her hands between cats?

For breeders and pet shops alike, the money to be made from selling cats depends on a fast turnover. The breeder knows that his kittens have the benefit of natural immunity for the first eight to twelve weeks of life while they are being nursed and shortly afterward.

As long as he sells the cat during the brief immune period after the cat has been weaned, the dealer is home free, health-wise. But if the kitten hangs around the breeder's place or a pet shop, it's likely to catch something—particularly an upper-respiratory infection, to which young cats are especially susceptible. Once a shop owner has to start paying vet bills for a sick kitten, he has lost money, so his aim is to sell them young and quickly, naturally enough.

This take-'em-young, sell-'em-fast kitten movement is all a sad, pathetic human business that cats are caught up in, and they are the only sufferers, unless you think the person foolish enough to spend two or three hundred dollars for some special cat is suffering. I don't.

I'm not saying that all cats are the same and that any cat will do for any owner. I am saying that the cat you love is the best cat in the whole world whether he has long, short, or no hair at all. However, loving a cat is not enough. There are some facts you should know or try to find out about the new pet you are bringing into your home.

Certainly, no one should acquire a kitten less than ten weeks old regardless of where it comes from. Can you judge the age of your kitten? Can you find out with some certainty how old he is?

Every effort should be made to get the medical history or some facts about where the cat came from, whether it was a stray, from a private home, or wherever. The more you know of a cat's recent origin the better prepared you are to care for it.

Some very important things you will want to know are:
1. Was the cat in contact with other cats?
2. What was he fed?
3. Did he have any prophylactic injections?
4. Has he shown any symptoms of illness?

Asking the right questions does not mean that you are going to get honest answers, but you should try for them. In any event, acquiring a new cat is always a gamble.

For the record, cats fall into three classifications:
1. Common domestics, the alley cats, form the biggest group. They're a little bit of everything all mixed up together. The

common domestics are usually short-haired. Even if they are half or three-quarters common domestic, they are not going to have very long hair.

2. Pedigreed short-haired cats make up the next classification. It's a large one, and the cats in this category are classified by breed—Siamese, Burmese, Abyssinians and so forth. Currently, the Siamese is the most popular cat in this classification. I think part of the reason is talkativeness. The older one gets, the more it talks, much like elderly people who go around muttering to themselves night and day.

3. The last classification comprises long-haired cats, and they are categorized by color—red tabby, white, blue, etc. Tabby just means that the fur has lines.

I haven't mentioned the Maine Coon cat which is supposed to be a cross between raccoons and wild house cats. It just ain't so. They're nice, big cats, and that's all.

Today, 85 percent of my work is with common domestics, 10 percent with pedigreed shorthairs, and 5 percent with long-haired cats. Long-haired cats used to be more popular than they are today, and I think the reason for the decline is the care they require. They've got to be combed and brushed daily. But even when that is done religiously, a longhair can still end up with painfully matted fur and have to be shaved.

I have treated some extreme cases of matting where I had to anesthetize the longhair and shave off its entire coat. It would come off in one long piece, like a horse's saddle blanket. More often than not, I try to avoid such drastic measures and just scissor-cut what I have to.

Cat fur grows back completely within two to three months. A cat who has had his fur cut or shaved off may feel the cold for a while, but aside from that there is no damage to the animal, except to its vanity. And cats are vain creatures. I've seen cats try to hide after a haircut. And several times I've seen a shaved cat stop in front of a mirror and just stare at its reflection in confusion. The expression on the cat's face seems to be, "Who the hell is that?"

But vanity is no reason to spare a longhair who needs it from having his fur clipped. Knotted fur is both disturbing and painful to a cat. Furthermore, it is unhealthy. The knot starts on the ends of the hairs. The fur mats up behind the knot, and the skin is pulled as the matted mess gets closer and closer to the skin. Dandruff will accumulate beneath the matting where the cat can't clean, and the cat may develop dry skin and other irritations.

Even short-haired cats need brushing and combing to remove loose hairs and prevent hair balls that come from swallowing too much fur as they clean themselves.

When cats lived in the wild, they needed their heavy winter coats, which they shed in the summer. The summer coat, in turn, would be shed as the heavier winter fur grew in. But an apartment cat doesn't need its winter coat at all. In fact, apartment living with its controlled temperatures confuses Mother Nature's plans for cats entirely, and the result is year-round shedding, not just at seasonal intervals.

Some cats, rare ones I'll admit, come to love their daily grooming, especially those whose owners have made it a habit since kittenhood. The rarest of all cats that I have ever known in the cleanliness department has to be Mary Gangem's seal-point Siamese, Holly. Holly is probably the cleanest cat in Greenwich, and maybe in the entire state of Connecticut. Holly likes to be vacuumed!

If you've ever seen a cat in a room when a vacuum cleaner is turned on, you know that it runs as if the devil himself were after it. But not Holly. Aside from being a loving, quiet and gentle cat, Holly showed a marked fascination with Mary's Electrolux the first time she saw it in action.

Holly would never leave the room when Mary brought out the vacuum cleaner. Instead, Holly would slink around the room, working closer and closer to the machine. Then she'd play with the hose and cuddle up to the tank. The noise of the vacuum cleaner in action didn't frighten her at all. After a few minutes of romantic foreplay with the hose, Holly would flip herself over on her back next to the tank with her feet thrashing about in the air.

One day Mary had the small upholstery-brush attachment on, ready to clean the sofa, and there was Holly, on her back, in seductive invitation to the machine. Mary gently touched the brush attachment to Holly's fur so that the Siamese could see how it felt. Holly loved it! She stayed put and began to purr.

Mary knew a good thing when she saw it. She ran the brush attachment over Holly's body, and Holly flipped about so that Mary could vacuum all of her. When she came to Holly's tail, Mary removed the brush attachment, and let the end of the tail get sucked up by the hose nozzle.

I wouldn't have believed any of this if I had not seen Holly get a vacuuming. It turns out that Holly is not fussy about which attachment, if any, is used. She lies down and purrs whenever Mary goes to the closet where she keeps the vacuum cleaner, and if, by chance, Mary starts housecleaning without first giving Holly her beauty treatment, the house is filled with Siamese cat talk, and Mary runs the risk of having one of her nylons snagged by a cat claw.

Holly is certainly unique, so don't get carried away by her story and try to vacuum your cat. Chances are your cat will be like most of them and regard the vacuum cleaner as a mortal enemy. But if you should see old Oswilla sidling up to the vacuum cleaner with obvious interest, you might give her a try with one of the gentler brushes. It could solve your cat-grooming problem.

Back when they lived in Manhattan, Maurice Dolbier, who is today the book editor of the Providence *Journal*, had a long-haired cat named Drusus who had to be shaved. When I examined Drusus, I realized that his long fur had become so covered with tangles that I would have to denude him completely.

When Drusus regained consciousness at the Dolbiers' apartment, his half-sister, Jenny—same mother, different father—had no idea who he was. Drusus, still a little groggy from the anesthetic and not aware of what had happened to him, started across the room toward Jenny, with whom he shared a warm feline relationship. To his amazement, gentle, easygoing Jenny arched her back and hissed and spat at him. Drusus didn't know what was going on, and so he continued toward her. After all, he was her favorite brother. To his horror, Jenny slapped him across the nose.

Poor Drusus slunk away. From that moment on, he went into a deep depression. He hid himself from Jenny and the Dolbiers, and he refused to eat or be seen.

A few days later, with Drusus still in hiding, a friend of the Dolbiers arrived from Rhode Island, bringing Mary Dolbier several branches of sea lavender as a house gift. Mary took the branches into the kitchen and placed them on the kitchen counter, planning to arrange them later on. She rejoined her guest in the living room.

Drusus must have crept out of his hiding place and discovered the sea lavender, which attracted him like catnip.

When the Dolbiers went back into the kitchen, they discovered bits of sea lavender scattered all over the room. In the middle of the floor was Drusus, happy, hungry, and with a decided what-the-hell attitude toward Jenny, who was backed into a corner, hissing and confused.

Obviously, from his attitude, the sea lavender wreckage had to be Drusus's work, but the Dolbiers found it hard to believe that this weakened, undernourished cat had actually made the leap to the counter top. They took the remains of the lavender branches to the living room and placed them on the piano top, a higher jump. Then they shut Jenny up in one of the guest rooms with enough food and litter to get her through the night.

In the morning, they found sprigs of sea lavender all over the apartment, and Drusus, hairless but happy, asleep on top of the piano.

Leroy Lincoln was chairman of the board of Metropolitan Life Insurance, a busy, dynamic man. His wife, I knew, was mad about their four Siamese cats and one longhair, but I had no idea how Mr. Lincoln felt. He had never given me any indication that he cared beans about the cats, that is, until the longhair had to be shaved.

The long-haired cat had established himself as the dominant cat in the household, and he put up with no nonsense from the four Siamese.

The longhair insisted on dining alone, and only when he finished eating were the other cats allowed to get to their bowls. If one of the Siamese found a sleeping place that interested the longhair, he immediately booted it out of the place and settled himself in. At any time that a cat didn't behave to his satisfaction, the longhair had no hesitancy about going into action. The fights were brief and noisy, and they always ended with a Siamese slinking away in defeat.

The Lincolns lived in a twenty-room townhouse near the corner of 68th Street and Park Avenue. The five Lincoln cats had their own big room at the top of the house. The other upstairs rooms were the servants' quarters.

One day Mrs. Lincoln, accompanied by the chauffeur, who was carrying the longhair, came to my Park Avenue office. The longhair's fur was badly matted. Mrs. Lincoln explained that she was enroute to their Pennsylvania farm, but she didn't want to delay having the cat taken care of. Could I anesthetize him and clip his fur, and would it be possible for me to drop the cat back at the house, where someone would look after him? I said I would.

That afternoon, I anesthetized the cat and cut out the fur tangles. I left the sleeping cat with a ruff around the face and some fur around each of his ankles. He looked like a lion, which I thought suited his personality.

When I closed my office for the day, George Mosby put the sleeping cat in his carrier and took it out to my car. I drove to the Lincoln townhouse and gave the carrier to one of the servants, with instructions that the cat was to be kept isolated from the other four until he woke up, and that he was to be turned every two hours so that his lungs wouldn't get congested. My instructions were either forgotten or ignored.

I must have stopped to make a house call on my way home, because it was more than two hours later that I called my answering service to get my messages. There was one message that was repeated three times: "Call Mr. Lincoln."

By the time I reached him, Leroy Lincoln had worked himself into a lather. When he calmed down enough, he told me what had happened. The sleeping and clipped longhair had been taken upstairs and placed in the room with the four subservient Siamese. Mr. Lincoln came home shortly afterward and went up to his bedroom to change and take a nap. He had just about fallen asleep when a wild, screaming racket broke out over his head. He leaped from the bed and ran up to the cats' room.

Obviously, the four Siamese had sniffed around the sleeping stranger in their room for a while. Then they had recognized the odd-looking cat as their old enemy, the longhair. When they realized that he was out cold and couldn't defend himself, they ganged up on him.

"My favorite cat! My favorite cat!" Leroy Lincoln moaned over the telephone. "It's terrible. You've got to come over right away!"

"I'll get there as fast as I can," I said.

When Mr. Lincoln took me up to the cats' room, I found the four Siamese bunched in one corner looking very pleased with themselves, and the longhair, a beat-up mess, hunched up across the room, wondering what had happened to him.

I had to put twelve stitches in the longhair. Through the whole procedure Leroy Lincoln stood beside me muttering, "My favorite cat!" over and over to himself. I knew he cared deeply —at least about the longhair. I don't know for certain how he felt about the Siamese, but I'll bet he could cheerfully have strangled each of them at that moment.

This time the longhair, who had been put to sleep again while I was taking the stitches, was carried to the master bedroom to sleep off the anesthetic.

When the longhair was fully awake again and returned to the cats' room, the Siamese stayed as far away as possible from the boss of the room. The longhair was twice as tough with them as he had been before—the old order was restored with a vengeance.

Chapter 10

BECAUSE CATS ARE loners, rather aloof creatures, a whole lot of nonsense has been created about them and often an owner believes this bunkum. Especially in the area of food.

There isn't a day that goes by without some client telling me that his or her cat is a finicky eater and will only eat such-and-such, or he keeps the cat bowl filled to the brim because, as everyone knows, a cat will only eat when hungry. To both these statements, I say baloney!

Cats will eat almost anything from artichokes to olives. If the cat gets finicky, it is because it has an owner that can be bullied and buffaloed into giving it anything it wants. It is a rare owner who has the guts to give the cat what it should have and then sit tight for two or three days while the cat whines and rejects what is in its dish. If the owner holds out, he'll see the finicky cat turn into a hungry cat and eat its meal.

And as far as a cat eating only what its body needs, let me tell you a story.

Several years ago I received a telephone call from a client who was worried about her cat, who seemed to be getting lame. I said I would stop by.

I checked my records and realized that I hadn't seen the cat in a year and that it was time for its annual upper-respiratory shot.

When I arrived at the apartment, the butler opened the door for me and led me to the kitchen, where my patient was waiting. I was told that "the Madam" would be home shortly.

I looked around for my patient and found her sprawled under the table. What at first I thought was an orange fur rug moved slightly and I realized it was the cat, the fattest cat I had ever seen. I couldn't believe my eyes. The poor thing was as wide as it was long, and when I hoisted it up to stand on the table its belly scraped the tabletop.

I called the butler and asked him if he knew what the cat weighed. He said it weighed around twenty-eight pounds. When I asked who fed the cat, he said he did. "I give the cat a pound of freshly ground beef each day."

I found that hard to believe. A pound of beef every day is too much food for a cat, but it is not enough to cause such obesity.

The woman came home shortly after I'd started examining the cat, who was so sluggish it didn't even struggle in my hands. When I asked the woman about the cat's diet, she gave me the same answer that her butler had.

I couldn't understand it. I couldn't vouch for the butler's honesty but I knew the woman wouldn't lie to me. In a state of confusion I finished my examination of the huge orange blob and said I would come back the next day. The sight of that cat so upset me that I forgot to give it its shot.

I got a bad night's sleep that evening. That monster cat kept lumbering through my mind and waking me to worry how she had gotten that way.

I went back the next day. I told the butler he could leave me alone with the cat in the kitchen. I began by giving the cat her annual shot. When I went to toss out the disposable syringe I saw four empty cans of dog food in the garbage.

A light dawned. I knew that my client didn't own a dog, and I didn't think that people who could afford butlers ever ate dog food.

I called for the butler and asked him who was eating the stuff. He confessed that he was feeding the dog food to the cat without the owner's knowledge. Between the ground beef and the four cans of dog food, that cat was eating about five pounds of food each day!

I hit the roof. "You're killing that cat, do you know that? Why are you doing this?"

At first he didn't want to tell me. When I threatened to tell his employers, he confessed. He had read about an English cat that weighed thirty-three pounds, and he wanted this American cat to beat the record.

He begged me not to tell his employers and he promised to put the cat back on its hamburger-only diet, and to cut that back, too, to a smaller amount.

Within a week the cat showed signs of improvement and began to move around a little more actively. But it was too late for the poor thing. One day, the still way-overweight creature tried to jump up on a chair, but her weight was against her. She couldn't get airborne enough and she fell backward and broke her back. I had to put her to sleep.

So much for the myth that cats eat only what they need.

While we're at it, dogs are also notorious overeaters. Quite a few years ago, I had a call to see a dog belonging to a priest at a Catholic church in Westchester. Before I could even ring the bell, the door opened and the priest's housekeeper came out to tell me the cause of the dog's distress.

It was the priest, she said. He was in bed with the flu and he fed candy all day long to his beloved dog, and she couldn't get him to stop. Certainly with the father ill, she couldn't keep his dog away from him, so what could she do?

Armed with the information, I went up to the priest's room where I saw one of the worst-looking specimens of dog that ever met my eyes. It was a cocker spaniel, and it was almost square in shape. When it moved, its keel brushed the floor.

As soon as I entered the room, the priest motioned for me to close the door and come close to the bed, "so she won't hear us."

He pointed to the floor to indicate the housekeeper below. "Ever since I took sick that woman's been overfeeding the dog. Just look at him."

I felt as if I was caught in the middle of a family quarrel. When I saw the open box of candy on the night table beside his bed, I asked the priest if he liked candy.

"I eat a few pieces every day," he said.

"And does the dog like candy, too?"

The priest shrugged. "He's not especially keen on it."

During this conversation, I accidentally on purpose tapped the candy box. The dog immediately waddled over to me. I just looked at the priest for a minute. He blushed. Then I told him in no uncertain terms that candy was not for the dog. "If you love your dog, you must stop giving him chocolates, now and forever."

The priest promised he would. "But I assure you, Dr. Camuti, the problem isn't with me but that woman downstairs. You can find out for yourself if you'll just look in the kitchen garbage can to see the number of empty dog-food cans she has thrown in today."

When I went downstairs I asked to wash my hands in the kitchen. The housekeeper showed me the way. I dried my hands on a paper towel and asked where the garbage can was so I could throw away the used towel.

The priest was right. I saw twice the number of cans I should have.

I glared at the housekeeper. "You have the nerve to blame the father, and here you are feeding that poor dog enough food for two, maybe three dogs. Do you want to kill it?"

"I love that dog, I swear I do."

"Well, your love is going to send it to an early grave."

I told her what the correct amount of food for the dog was, and she promised to stick to it. Within a few months, the dog was back to his proper size. But at no time then or for as long as I saw the cocker spaniel did either party ever admit that he —or she—had done anything wrong. It was always the other one.

Assuming you have a normal, healthy cat—and if you don't, your veterinarian will prescribe a special diet—feeding your cat and keeping him healthy should be a fairly simple matter. Cats are carnivores. They eat meat. That's it in a nutshell.

Sure, cats love fish, but did you ever see a cat go fishing, outside of maybe trying to grab the goldfish out of the bowl? The answer is no, because cats weren't designed to be fishers. Most of them hate the water.

Cats are meat eaters, and in the country they go out after mice, moles and rabbits. Because those three tasty items are pretty scarce in most city apartments, I tell all my clients to feed their cats beef, and I suggest they buy baby-food beef, the kind that is pureed and put up for infants. I figure that if it is meant for babies, the stuff has got to be pure, without any of those "beef byproducts," whatever they are, in canned cat food. If you truly love your cat give him baby beef. That, and water in his dish is the best basic diet for a normal, healthy cat.

Liver and kidneys, promoted by cat-food manufacturers, are all right once in a while, but not with any great frequency. Organ meats are rich in certain ingredients and lacking in others.

Cats love chicken, turkey and other fowl, and they can certainly have that once in a while, but make sure there are no bones in what you serve Nicodemus and Oswilla. Cats in the wild catch birds and small animals but they don't eat the bones. They do, however, eat the contents of their catch's stomachs and get some grain and vegetation that way, so you might let your cat have some cooked vegetables with his dinner every now and then.

Keep in mind that a cat does not digest carbohydrates well. Starch digestion for us begins in our saliva, but a cat gulps down his food. He doesn't masticate his food because he has tearing teeth, not chewing teeth, and he doesn't have the same enzymes we do which are needed to break down certain foods.

A cat needs some fat in his diet, but not much. While many cats can tolerate a higher percentage of fat than 5 percent, I feel that 5 percent is adequate.

Information on the fat content, ash content, and just about any other content you can think of appears by law on every can of cat food, but it is difficult for the lay person to interpret. I think labels could be made much simpler with percentage listings that the buyer could easily understand.

Milk can be part of the cat's diet if it agrees with him. In the wild, a cat doesn't get milk after he is weaned. The milk that we humans drink can cause constipation or diarrhea in a cat. If this occurs with your cat, cut him off it immediately. Some people find success with a mixture of half water and half condensed milk.

Many people like to give their cats an occasional egg. Fine. Half a raw egg is good if the cat likes it. I've been told by some clients that they only give their cats the yolk of an egg because the white is high in ash, which causes urinary problems for male cats. Since the ash debate isn't settled as yet, I'd just as soon see a cat get half a whole egg. But again, only now and then.

Table scraps are every cat's favorite, but the owner should make it a treat, not a staple of the cat's diet. If you have had your cat in the kitchen while you are preparing a shrimp dish or hamburgers, you know he wants some. He can have a little bit, but only once in a while.

People are always asking me if it's all right for their cats to have stuffed olives—"Boobie is wild about them, Doctor," or cantaloupe, or potato chips or chocolate chip cookies. My rule of thumb is that anything your cat keeps down is fine—once in a while. Just don't let him have it as a regular food, and certainly don't encourage or tolerate thievery from the snack platter or the dining table.

I know of one rather well-known New York hostess who lost a few good friends when she insisted that her cat be allowed to stay on the table during a dinner party. I heard about her through a client of mine who went to her house one night with his wife and found his hostess's tabby facing him on the dining table with definite designs on his dish. When my client protested, the hostess just brushed it aside. "He likes to be there," she explained.

"We have two cats of our own and they are never allowed on the dining table," my client said.

The hostess smiled. "Mine is."

"It's either the cats or us," my client said.

"The cat stays."

My client and his wife got up and left.

Another noted hostess, whose friends are more permissive, also allows her white Angora to sit on the table at her dinners. But her Angora often provides some entertainment when he sets the tip of his tail on fire as he waves it while strolling past the dinner candles. The cat usually leaves the table for the remainder of the evening after a guest extinguishes him with water or wine.

As to how often a cat should be fed, it depends on the routine of the household. Generally, twice a day—morning and evening —is best. That way the cat is being fed approximately every twelve hours and isn't going too long without food.

In some households where the clients have midnight snacks the cat gets one, too. The number of times a day that the cat eats doesn't matter, so long as you divide the food he gets into portions that add up to a sensible amount for the entire day. If your cat requires a can or a can and a half of cat food a day, then he should get a jar or a jar and a half of baby, or junior, beef. I'm not saying the cat will be happy with this, especially if he has been spoiled by loving but foolish owners, but he will be a lot healthier. In my time I've heard of cats who loved leftover stew, meaty spaghetti sauce, ice cream—if you must give ice cream to your cat, wait until it melts, as cold isn't good for cats—and corn on the cob.

The trick in a healthy diet for your cat is never one of finding a food your cat likes. It is sticking to what you know is good for your cat. The problem arises when the cat passes up its regular diet and holds out for liver or fish (those urinary stones that male cats sometimes develop are largely phosphates, and fish is high in phosphate) or some special dish you let him have once in a while. This is the moment when too many cats become spoiled animals and owners their servants. I'll admit it's difficult not to give in when your beloved cat starts crying and rubbing against your leg and refusing to touch its food. The cat isn't starving, but deliberately manipulating you. I've never yet seen a house cat commit suicide by starving itself to death, and I don't expect to. When that cat is hungry enough it will eat what you give it with gusto. Better still, it will know who is the boss.

I had a client who just couldn't break her cat, Alfie, of the all-liver diet she had started him on. At least, that's what she said. What I thought was that she didn't have the guts for a show-down with Alfie. And poor Alfie was a listless, burned-out cat at the age of twelve from his limited diet. Luckily the lady got transferred to a big job in Atlanta, and she left Alfie with friends while she went South to find an apartment. Her friends turned out to be made of stronger stuff than she, and they stood up to Alfie. By the time his mistress sent for him, Alfie was weaned away from liver and eating his baby beef gratefully. He arrived in Atlanta a much friskier cat.

I still have a note I received from a couple who moved from the city to their summer home near Yonkers. I couldn't believe it. They wrote to tell me that their cats didn't like Westchester water so they were bringing up jars of city water for the cats each weekend. I grabbed the phone the minute I finished the letter. "Are you crazy? Where do you think city water comes from? Westchester, that's where!"

In terms of cats and what they will and will not eat, I think the word "finicky" is one that only cat owners use. Every veterinarian knows how unfinicky an eater a cat can be. It is a rare year that goes by for me that I don't see at least one cat that has swallowed a needle and thread or one of those plastic-coated metal ties that come on the ends of packaged bread. There are too many cat toys on the market that are dangerous, too many things around the home that can fascinate a cat and end up in its stomach. The Tree House Animal Foundation of Chicago has published a list entitled, "Household Dangers To Cats" and they have allowed me to reprint it. You'll find it at the end of this chapter. I hope you'll read it. I wish some of my clients had.

Boris Brasol was a writer of legal texts and a great cat lover. In fact, he said he couldn't work unless his cat was on his desk.

One Christmas, he and his wife decided to go away for the holidays, and they arranged for their cat to board with me at Mount Vernon. To make the cat feel more at home during its stay with me, they brought some Christmas cards and other holiday decorations. I didn't mind them stringing Christmas cards around the outside of his cage, though I thought it was foolish, but I did object when they brought in a tiny Christmas tree to put inside his cage. "Now, look," I said, "the cards are one thing, but Christmas trees are not good for cats. It could poison him."

The Brasols brushed that aside. "He won't eat it, you'll see. We have a tree every year and he never bothers with it."

I warned them that if they insisted on putting the tiny tree inside the cage I wouldn't be responsible. I might as well have been talking a foreign language for all they listened to me. They felt so guilty about leaving their cat behind that they just had to give him a tree.

Sure enough, the cat ate some of the tree needles and died of turpentine poisoning. I felt very badly when I told the Brasols —but I had warned them.

I'll never forget the Sunday morning call I got from an hysterical woman, a maid who had been left in charge of the cat at the Park Avenue apartment of Paul Kent, a stockbroker, while he was in Europe. "Come quick, Dr. Camuti, the cat's intestines are coming out the back end."

I got out my car and raced right over. When I got there, I could see that the maid was right, up to a point. There was something sticking out from under the cat's tail, but I knew it wasn't a prolapsed rectum.

It was cord. About an inch of it was hanging out. There was no way to guess how much more there was inside the cat.

I decided to take quick action. I scooped up the cat and put it on the piano. With one hand I grabbed the inch of rope. With the other I gave the cat a hefty swat across the rump. The cat went flying across the room, and twenty-four inches of rope came out of its rectum. It was a window sash!

But the maid didn't know that. She screamed, "He's pulling out the intestines!" and collapsed on the floor. The cat was fine but it took me half an hour to bring the maid around.

Walter Millis, an editorial writer, and his wife, also a journalist, lived at the Dakota on Central Park West with their cats. One day, one of the cats started playing with an electric cord, bit into it and got a terrible electric shock and burn. Not only did the skin break down, but also part of the muscle so that a portion of the bony structure of the mouth was exposed on the left side of the face. Luckily, the Millises were home and they telephoned me immediately.

When I saw the cat, I thought it didn't have a prayer. I suggested putting it to sleep, but the Millises were determined to save their beloved pet, so we went to work. Or they did, under my guidance.

I saw the cat every day, but Mr. and Mrs. Millis tended to it around the clock. They took shifts keeping the jaw clean while the wound was fresh so infection wouldn't set in, and they spoon-fed liquids into the battered mouth.

Each time I went up to their apartment, I expected them to tell me that the cat had died. When the cat was still alive by the end of the second week, I too began to hope. Through all this, the cat just lay in the little bed they had fixed up for him padded with Mrs. Millis's old bathrobe, a longtime favorite of the cat's for napping.

In the early weeks of treatment I told Mr. and Mrs. Millis that they would have to massage the cat and turn it periodically to keep its circulation going if they hoped to save it. Despite their busy lives, they added those duties to the mouth swabbings and the spoon-feedings without complaint.

After a month went by, I told them I thought the cat was out of danger. And then one day, Mrs. Millis called me at my office to tell me the cat had purred for the first time. I nearly burst into tears.

Eventually, the cat was able to eat and run around again, but its face never fully healed, and you could always see the uncovered lower jaw and teeth on the left side.

As for the long hours and weeks they had spent to save the cat's life, Mrs. Millis summed it all up when she said, "It was easy. We love him."

I think I have made my point that cats will eat almost anything that strikes their fancy. They are not finicky. It is their owners who are foolish and give in to them and lose the upper hand.

Of all the spoiled cats I have ever met, I think Bunker, a Siamese, takes the cake. He belonged to a client I had in the late '30s and early '40s. She was a sensible lady in all areas of her life except where Bunker was concerned. By the time I met Bunker, he had been spoiled rotten.

It wasn't bad enough that the cat lived on an exclusive diet of canned crabmeat, but his mistress had spoiled him to the point that just any old crabmeat would not do. He ate only Japanese crabmeat.

That his diet was more expensive than most cats' was no great hardship for his owner. She was well paid as an investment advisor for Columbia University. What turned her foolish indulgence of her cat into a problem was World War II. Shortly after the Japanese attack on Pearl Harbor and the declaration of war against Japan, Japanese crabmeat became hard to find. And Bunker could tell the difference between Japanese crabmeat and domestic brands. On the latter, he just turned his back and walked away.

Since Columbia University is uptown and the lady lived downtown she began covering quite a large part of the city tracking down Bunker's dinner. Delicatessen owners all over the city took to looking at her suspiciously when she asked for Japanese crabmeat. Occasionally she found a store that had a case of it they had taken off the shelf and she would buy all of it that she could. But as the war progressed, the crabmeat became harder and harder to find.

"Give him something else and just wait for him to get hungry enough," I told her. "He'll learn that he's got to eat what you give him."

She shook her head. "You don't understand. I couldn't do that. I love him too much. Besides, he won't let me sleep at night when I've tried that. He just sits on my bed howling for crabmeat. I located one can the other day and gave him half of it that evening. I thought I'd save the rest for the next day. But Bunker knew it was in the refrigerator. He kept running back and forth from me to the kitchen yowling and scolding. I had to give it to him."

One lucky day, she located a market with several cans of Japanese crabmeat on the shelf. She took them all and asked the proprietor if he had any more. He said he did.

When she said she'd take them all, he got suspicious. "Are you selling this on the black market, lady?"

"Oh, no," she said, but she couldn't bring herself to admit the crabmeat was for her cat. "It's for a friend of mine. I wouldn't dream of selling it."

The storekeeper seemed to sense that there was something funny going on, and he refused to sell her his supply. He even took back some of the cans she had taken from the shelf. "No hoarding," he said. "Two should hold you for awhile. You come back when you need more and I'll have it for you."

She was thrilled to get the two cans for Bunker, and to know that the shopkeeper had more. She prayed he had an enormous supply. Though his shop was way out of her way on her return from Columbia to her apartment she went there every other day for her allotted two cans.

"You really like that stuff," the store owner said one day.

"Oh, it's not for me. I told you. It's for my friend."

"A Japanese?" he said casually.

"No—er—a Siamese," she said and left quickly.

123

Two days later when she returned, she noticed a policeman loitering at the doorway.

The storekeeper gave her a big wave of the hand as she entered. "Here for your Japanese crabmeat?" he said in a loud voice.

"Yes." She noticed the policeman come inside the store.

The storekeeper took his time putting her two cans of crabmeat into a bag. Though she didn't turn to look, she was certain that the policeman was studying her.

"Who did you say these were for?" the storekeeper asked. "A Japanese friend?"

"Not Japanese. Siamese."

"Where does he live?"

"With me," she said, feeling herself growing flustered and angry at the same time.

But the grocer persisted. "When did he come to this country?"

She was torn between her desire to tell the man she didn't have to answer his questions and her fear of cutting herself off from the supply of crabmeat for Bunker. "He was born here," she said.

"A Nisei, huh?"

That was the final straw. "Look," she said, "we're talking about a cat. A Siamese cat, not a person."

"Really?" the man said, and she could tell that he didn't believe her. "You go to all this expense and trouble for a cat?"

"Yes, I do," she said and put her money on the counter and grabbed the bag from the storekeeper and fled. Though she didn't look back, she was fairly certain that the policeman was following her.

She never saw anyone suspicious, but for several weeks afterward she was certain that she was followed.

The ridiculousness of the situation brought home to the woman how far overboard she had gone in her subservience to her cat. If she was being suspected of being an enemy agent by her country all because of Bunker, then it was time to really do something about his appetite.

124

And what did she do? She weaned him away from Japanese crabmeat and onto homemade pâté.

She told me that so-called happy bit of news when I was giving Bunker his annual distemper shot. "Well, aren't you proud of me?" she asked.

I stared at her. "Whatever you do," I said, "don't let him taste caviar."

HOUSEHOLD DANGERS TO CATS

Many ordinary, harmless-looking objects in your house can spell danger for your cat.

1. *Tinfoil, Corks, etc.*
Cats may love to play with a tinfoil ball or a cork on a string, but these objects can kill. If lodged in the throat, your cat could strangle; if chewed or partially eaten they can cause intestinal blockage. Keep tinfoil, corks, and other such objects away from your cat. Cellophane wrappers (on cigarette packages) can turn "glassy" in your cat's stomach and cause a painful death.

2. *Strings, Yarn, etc.*
Never leave a cat alone with string or yarn. These are easily swallowed and can cause strangulation, intestinal blockage or even death. One local veterinarian has seen many deaths from cats eating the string some beef roasts are tied up with. And don't be fooled by the silly stereotype of a kitten playing with a ball of yarn—don't take a chance with your pet's life.

3. *Rubber Bands*
Cats love to tug on rubber bands—but any size rubber band is dangerous and can be fatal if swallowed. (If swallowed whole, they can wrap around intestines much like string and yarn.) A

safe policy is to keep rubber bands in a drawer or container where your cat won't see or find them.

4. *Poisonous Plants*

Poinsettias are particularly deadly, as are azaleas and the dieffenbachia (dumb cane). The dumb cane is well named, for it can actually paralyze your cat's mouth. Other plants to avoid are philodendron, ivy, chrysanthemums, castor bean, mistletoe (berries especially), rhubarb (leaves), buttercups, cherry (twigs, leaves, bark, fruit stones), daffodil (bulbs), daphne (berries), iris (leaves, roots, and fleshy parts), jonquil (bulbs), poison ivy, privet, lily-of-the-valley (leaves, flowers, roots), mushrooms, narcissus (bulbs), star of Bethlehem (bulb), oak (acorns, young shoots and leaves), oleander, sumac, sweet pea (seeds and pods), rosary pea (shiny red and black seeds), potatoes (especially the eye and any sprouts from the eye; the "potato" as we cook it is okay), apricot and peach (pits). (For a complete listing of dangerous plants, consult your librarian or your veterinarian.)

5. *Cleaning Fluids, Rodent & Bug Killers*

Although most cats avoid chemicals because of their smell, there is always a chance your cat will take an experimental taste. One lick can be fatal. As with children, keep all chemicals, paints, poisons, cleaning fluids, etc., tightly capped and out of reach. Do not use bug killer in powder form—your cat could walk through it and lick his paws. Do not use "roach cakes" or other edible killing tablets. If a cat toy should come into contact with insecticide, throw it away immediately—poison can retain its killing power for indefinite periods of time. Death by poison can be slow and excruciating.

A good professional exterminator can help you rid your home or apartment of bugs or rodents with a minimum of danger to your cat. *Tell him you have a cat.* Then remove your pet and his food/water dishes from the house during spraying and until all rooms are aired out afterwards. Do not believe manufacturer claims that there is no danger to a cat from their poison or product. There can be.

More poisons: *Phenol:* Check bottles for combinations of words having phenol in the spelling. Examples of phenol products: Lysol, some mouth washes, calamine lotion, soaps and detergents containing hexachlorophene. *Coal Tar Products:* Pine Sol and Tegrin are two common examples. *Acids and Bases:* Hydrochloric acid, sulfuric acid, battery acid, lye, bleaches (including powdered and Clorox) and ammonia. *Miscellaneous:* Crayons, lime fertilizers, broken fluorescent bulbs, furniture polish, cloth dyes, paint and varnish remover, dishwashing compounds.

6. *Medicines*
Many people think medicine for people is good for cats, too. *This is not true.* Never give a cat any aspirin, even children's strength. This is deadly. All medicine should be kept in tightly closed containers and out of reach of your cat. Stilbestrol, benzyl benzoate, vitamins, tranquilizers and any other medicine can be fatal for a cat. Never administer any medicines or "home remedies" to your pet—consult your veterinarian if your pet is sick. If any medicine should be prescribed, he will do so. Follow directions closely on any prescription he might give you.

7. *Sharp Objects*
Keep all scissors, knives, straight pins, safety pins, razor blades, etc., stored securely away from your cat's reach. Puncture wounds can occur if your cat jumps onto a place where you've left a sharp object. Don't let your cat play with empty thread spools, either—chewing on the wood or plastic can put a splinter in your cat's mouth.

DANGEROUS CAT TOYS

Avoid any cat toy that is not well constructed. Never let a cat play with a toy that has glued-on decorations or trim. "Clowns" and "mice" are notorious for glued-on eyes, noses, tails, etc. These can come loose during play and be lodged in your cat's throat. Jingle bells are great fun, but be certain they are securely *tied* onto the toy, not just looped or glued on. If a jingle bell should come apart, dispose of all parts of it immediately (the edges are often sharp). Never let a cat play with a single jingle bell or any object so small it is easily swallowed.

Many toys sold in pet shops and supermarkets are hazardous. Check the toy for sturdiness before you buy.

Yarn toys should be avoided in general. Unless they are most securely braided or tied, they can come apart, tangle, and even choke a cat while he is playing with them.

GOOD, SAFE CAT TOYS

The best toys are *sewn* together, not glued—so they can take a lot of tossing around and biting without coming apart. Some of the knitted or crocheted balls sold by local animal groups are safe—they are best when stuffed with nylon stockings and do not have loops or strings attached.

Some household items are great for cats—many cats delight in "fighting" with the round cardboard tube or strip from an ordinary coathanger—the kind you would hang slacks over to avoid creasing. Ping-Pong balls are also easy to scoot around and difficult to hurt. In general, any soft toy that is well-constructed with no sharp corners or decorations, is fine. And the more lightweight they are, the better for pushing across the floor, tossing in the air and chasing after.

Remember: Your cat cannot judge safety for himself. He needs your help in selecting toys that are safe as well as fun!
　　　　　　　—TREE HOUSE ANIMAL FOUNDATION, Inc.
　　　　　　P.O. Box 11174 Chicago, Illinois 60611

Chapter II

WHEN I TELL PEOPLE that I make house calls for cats in New York City, I usually get a look that says I'm bluffing or I'm crazy. I can't say that I blame the person, but that look always catches me by surprise and makes me see my life from outside myself. I suppose what I do is sort of wacky, but I've been at it so long now that it has become natural to me and quite normal.

Luckily, most people never ask questions beyond the astonished "You mean you go to the cat instead of the cat coming to you?" The picture, I suppose, is that old Camuti may sometimes have a little trouble in finding the address or a place to park, but that's it.

If only it were as simple as that. I suppose it would be if all of my clients stayed in the same place year after year—which they don't—and if they didn't take their cats with them—which they do. And it would also help if they all lived in buildings with elevators or at least on the ground floor of walkups—which they don't.

One of the difficulties with growing older is that stairs have become a problem for me. And a heart attack several years ago has forced me to make it a policy not to climb any stairs beyond the second floor. Cats living above that have to come down to me.

I thought that when I started telling clients my new stair policy they'd hang up on me and find another veterinarian. I've had enough people through the years tell me I am not the most charming man in the world—and there are days when Alex agrees with them. Surprisingly enough, I didn't lose many clients at all. What happened instead is that I started treating cats in hallways and stairwells all over the city.

I can't say that a hallway or a stairwell is the ideal examining room, but it's not too bad, especially if there is an old-fashioned covered radiator there. It's usually the right height and width for my purpose, and the cats like the warmth in the winter. If it gets too warm, I tell the client to fetch some towels or newspapers to put on the radiator cover.

Sometimes these hallway meetings take on a carnival air, with people coming in or out of the building and stopping to find out what's going on, or neighbors gathering to peek over my shoulder. My cat patients don't like this any more than I do, so I try to convince my upstairs clients if at all possible to make friends with someone on a lower floor who will open his or her apartment for the examination. If nothing else, the lighting is better inside an apartment.

Nelly Quinn, who lived on the fifth floor of a West Side walkup called me because she thought her cat had ringworm. I reminded her that I could no longer make the climb to her apartment. Could she arrange to use a downstairs neighbor's apartment? She said she would try.

I told her that if we had to use the downstairs hallway as we had the last time I had seen her Mouser, a black-and-white domestic shorthair, she would have to make certain there was an electrical outlet because I would have to examine the cat with an ultraviolet light with a Woods filter. Miss Quinn told me she would work it all out.

When I arrived at her building, she told me through the intercom to wait for her at the foot of the stairs. Then she buzzed me into the building.

I found myself waiting in a drafty, smelly hallway for what

seemed like forever. I kept hearing footsteps coming down the stairs, but Nelly Quinn never seemed to arrive.

Finally, I saw her and a friend on the floor above. She was plugging extension cords into each other and working her way down five flights of stairs. Her friend was holding a snarl of cords and handing one after another to Nelly.

Eventually she reached me. Despite the cold in the hall, her face gleamed with perspiration. "What a job," she said. "I borrowed extension cords from every single person I know!"

While Nelly caught her breath, I plugged in my Woods light. To my surprise, it worked through that maze of extension cords. Nelly went back upstairs to fetch Mouser. Of course, after all that work on her part, Mouser didn't have ringworm.

Another upstairs client of mine was a couple who lived on 11th Street. They kept eight cats in their fourth-floor apartment. One of them caught a respiratory infection and passed it on to the other seven. I had to see them all daily for a month. It meant a great deal of going up and down stairs for the couple, but their ground-floor hallway was a pretty good setup for me. There was a radiator with a cover long enough and broad enough to serve as a medical table. Next to the radiator was an electrical outlet into which we plugged a hot plate for the pot of boiling water I needed (this was back before disposable syringes), and there was a bathroom under the stairs where I could wash my hands between cats.

The only problem was that the two apartments on the ground floor were being used as psychiatrists' offices. My clients hadn't said anything to the psychiatrists—only one of whom they knew —about my visit. Therefore the doctors hadn't said anything to their patients.

The first encounter between psychiatric patient and cat doctor took place when I was waiting in the hallway between cats, with my back to the wall, holding a syringe. The patient entered the building, took one look at me holding the needle, turned and ran back out. Other patients would press flat against the wall and inch down it to the doctor's office, eyes always on me, and pop into the office white-faced.

One night, a woman who had been in with her psychiatrist before I arrived, came out of the office and froze at the sight of me. Before I could say anything, she dashed into the bathroom, because, I assume, it was nearer than the front door. To make me think she was using the john instead of hiding from the mad doctor in the hall, she kept flushing the toilet. I can't say for certain how long she was in there, but I know I saw and treated two cats while she was still flushing.

Finally one of the psychiatrists heard all the water and came out to see what was the matter. Naturally, I was alone at the time.

He looked at me, at the boiling pot, at the towel on the radiator and asked what I was doing. "I'm treating some cats," I explained.

"Oh," he said very calmly, "really?"

"They're upstairs right now," I said.

"Oh," he said again, and stepped back into his office and locked the door. I think he assumed I was a patient of the other doctor on the floor.

As for the flushing lady, I hope she came out after I left.

About three weeks later, one of the psychiatrists went on vacation. My clients must have told him what we were up to, because he gave them the keys to his office. I was able to treat the eight cats on the psychiatrist's couch—another first for veterinary medicine, so far as I know.

Of course, it isn't always hallways. I had one client who used to sail his cat to me. Franklin Gregory, a columnist for the Newark *Star Ledger,* spent a great deal of time on his boat with his cat, who loved sailing as much as he did. Whenever the cat would take ill on a trip, he'd sail into City Island where I'd meet him and tend to his cat on board ship.

Dr. Clifford Baker, a radiologist, also had a sailing cat, but when she became ill the Bakers were too far away and I had to treat his Winkie-Pooh by telephone.

Winkie-Pooh, a Siamese, was an accomplished weekend sailor by the time she was three. In fact, Winkie-Pooh was so seaworthy a cat that the Bakers decided to take her along on their vacation trip to Maine aboard their thirty-two foot auxiliary sailboat, the Bali Hai.

It was an easy sail from their home port of Larchmont through Long Island Sound. But things roughened up on the twelve-hour sail to Edgartown, Massachusetts. They arrived, exhausted, and just as they passed Chappaquiddick Island, a July Fourth fireworks display went off from a point only a few yards away. The noise on deck was deafening, and bits of hazardous parachute flares rained down on them. Winkie-Pooh, already worn out from the long day, became so agitated that she had to be locked up in the lavatory.

She wasn't released until the ship rode at anchor and all was quiet again. Winkie-Pooh came slowly on deck. She seemed very subdued.

The next day's destination was Nantucket, twenty-eight miles farther east, so the Bakers lifted anchor early in the morning. Once out in the open, they again hit rough water.

Winkie-Pooh became depressed and lethargic and refused to eat, drink or stay up on deck. She hid below and moped. At first, after they arrived at Nantucket, Dr. Baker wasn't too concerned when Winkie-Pooh didn't snap back. He decided she just needed a rest and then she'd be fine. But within two days, Winkie-Pooh was visibly worse. She had stretched out on her side and seemed almost comatose. More alarming was the fact that she was breathing rapidly and there was foam running out of the side of her mouth.

The minute Dr. Baker saw the foam, he went ashore in search of a local veterinarian. He felt that the cat's condition was critical. Unable to find a veterinarian on the island, he called me in New York and described Winkie-Pooh's symptoms over the telephone. Being a physician himself, his observations were both acute and helpful to me.

"Do you have a hypodermic aboard?" I asked.

"No," he answered.

"Well, get one." I prescribed a medication I no longer remember. I said, "give her a hundred-milligram dose between the shoulders every hour until she shows signs of improvement. And call me if you have any questions. In fact, even if you don't have any questions, call me in a few hours and let me know how she's doing."

Dr. Baker made me repeat the dosage. He couldn't believe it. What I'd prescribed was the dosage you'd give to an adult on a weekly basis, not hourly to a moribund eight-pound cat. But even though he was skeptical, he agreed to follow my instructions.

He made a beeline for the nearest drugstore, where the druggist at first refused to sell him a syringe and needles. He was certain that the doctor was a drug addict. And, of course, Dr. Baker, being on vacation, hadn't brought his credentials along. After a lot of explaining about his background and the condition of his cat, he was able to buy what he needed and get back to Winkie-Pooh.

He administered the first shot exactly as I had told him to, then watched over the cat, waiting for signs of change. He was certain that I had made a dreadful error.

There was no change after the first shot, and he felt that Winkie-Pooh was not long for this world.

At the end of the hour, he administered the second shot. He couldn't believe his eyes—Winkie-Pooh was trying to get up on her feet. She wanted to get to her water bowl. He pulled it to her.

Before the next shot, she had drunk some water and was standing without assistance. Hour by hour, Dr. Baker and his wife watched their cat literally snap back to life.

Dr. Baker telephoned me as he said he would, still disbelieving the treatment even though he had administered it himself.

Winkie-Pooh was fully recovered in a few days, ready to resume her vacation. Dr. Baker made it a point of stopping in port every evening to telephone me with a report on the cat's progress. To this day, Dr. Baker finds it difficult to believe that the heavy dosage I prescribed didn't kill the cat.

The patient I probably saw more of than any other was Mary Henle's cat, Guapo—the same Guapo who had been smuggled in to see me in a pillowcase when I was in the hospital having my allergy tests. The reason is that Guapo lived longer than any cat I've ever known—twenty-one and a half years!

Mary and I became very close over the many years I saw Guapo. So close, in fact, that I've been made a cousin. My name is now Louis Joseph Henle Camuti, and Alex and I go to the annual Henle family parties.

Guapo was getting the combination of hormone and vitamin shots which make up my geriatric treatment for cats. Unfortunately, this is a procedure that all cat owners are not ready to understand or to pay for.

I start treatment when a cat reaches middle age—about nine or ten years—if the cat starts showing signs of slowing down. At this point, he may drink more water than he ever did before, his bowel movements may become disorganized, and he'll just seem to move and respond more slowly. I start his geriatric shots two or three times per week, for weeks at a time once a year.

When the cat reaches the next stage, about fourteen to sixteen years of age, I give him the treatments twice a year. After eighteen or nineteen, I may give him his shots every few months, and after that, it may go on almost continuously.

As I've said, not many people are willing to go through with this because it is expensive. But those who do and see the way the cats respond usually wish they could get the shots themselves.

Guapo's geriatric treatments began in September of his eleventh year. Shortly after I began the series, Mary became a guest lecturer at the Harvard Center for Cognitive Studies. Needless to say, it was a bit more difficult to get to Guapo in Cambridge than it was to reach Mary's 12th Street apartment.

Sometimes I went up to Cambridge, but I drew the line at

making the run three times a week, so Mary alternated with me and would drive Guapo down to New York City. Other times, we met in the middle, in Hartford, at my daughter-in-law's parents' home. With the kind of mileage both Mary and I were logging, Guapo ended his first series of geriatric shots looking better than either one of us.

I might have broken all records for mileage covered by a veterinarian in the line of duty if I had been able to answer in the affirmative to the wire I received from Charlotte and Joseph Kesselring—he wrote the play *Arsenic and Old Lace.*

FIDDLE ILL. CAN YOU COME? PLEASE PHONE
IMMEDIATELY. HOTEL EXCELSIOR NAPLES. UNABLE TO
GET YOU ON PHONE.

CHARLOTTE KESSELRING

I had to read the telegram twice to make certain it wasn't from Naples, Florida, instead of Naples, Italy. I knew that the Kesselrings were two of the most devoted cat people I had ever had as clients, but this request to fly to Italy for a sick cat was almost beyond belief. And Fiddle wasn't anything special, just an ordinary gray-and-white cat, one of many the Kesselrings had, but their favorite. The others stayed at their place in Woodstock, while Fiddle went everywhere with them.

I called Charlotte in Italy and had her describe Fiddle's symptoms—a general stoppage of all her plumbing. I suggested a course of treatment and told Charlotte to call me the next day.

I told her that the idea of my coming over was probably out of the question. I had just gotten out of the hospital after my heart attack, and I doubted that my doctor would let me make the trip.

Charlotte immediately said, "Have your doctor come, too. We'll pay for him as well."

I told her I'd check it out with my physician, and she said she would call me the next day.

As soon as I hung up, I called the airlines to check on flights —I liked the idea of seeing my ancestral homeland again. Then I called my internist, Dr. John Prutting.

He couldn't believe that I was even considering flying to Naples for a cat that couldn't urinate or move its bowels. When I told him that I was indeed thinking of going, he said, "You call Dr. Kwit first."

Dr. Kwit was my cardiologist and a top man in his field. I reached him at home. I had gotten about halfway through my reasons for wanting to make the trip when he cut in. "Wait a minute. My wife's got to hear this or she'll never believe me."

I heard him call to his wife to pick up the extension. Then he told me to start the whole thing over again. When I finished, there was a long silence. Finally, Dr. Kwit said, "I'm told I'm fairly important in my field, but as important as I've been, I have never had anyone call me to go to Europe, and here's Louis being asked over for a cat."

He said the whole idea was too risky for me so soon out of the hospital. He didn't change his mind when I told him that the Kesselrings had invited him, too.

Just for the hell of it, Dr. Kwit and I figured out what our time and all the expenses of a forty-eight hour trip to treat Fiddle would cost the Kesselrings. It came to approximately $7,000.

The next day, another cablegram arrived from Naples:

GOOD PROGRESS. BOTH NECESSARY MOVEMENTS.
STAYING NAPLES UNTIL SATURDAY. WILL NOT
TELEPHONE UNLESS EMERGENCY. WRITE US HOW YOU
ARE. HOTEL EXCELSIOR ROME.
CHARLOTTE KESSELRING

And that was the end of that. Fiddle had buried my European trip in her kitty litter!

Certainly, no trip before or since can touch my almost-house call to Italy, but one of the favorite places in which I have practiced veterinary medicine is an internists's office, the internist being my friend and doctor, John Prutting.

It all began when a patient of Dr. Prutting's came in for her annual checkup. While he examined her, she told him of her complaints and woes, most of them nonmedical. She was a book editor, divorced, with two children, and she'd recently lost her job. On top of that, her cat had broken its leg. The woman was concerned about spending the twenty-five dollars the Animal Medical Center would charge for X-raying the cat's leg. They had done an excellent job of setting the fracture, but she hated to spend twenty-five dollars to be told the leg was healing nicely and when to come in to have the wire removed that was holding the break in healing position.

Dr. Prutting, a cat lover himself, offered to help the lady out. He figured that a cat's leg would be only slightly larger than a human finger, no problem at all for his X-ray equipment. Since his X-ray technician was another cat lover, Dr. Prutting told the woman to bring her cat in and they'd X-ray the leg without charge.

On the appointed day the woman returned with her cat. The waiting room was filled, but the minute she entered, Dr. Prutting's nurse swooped down on her. "You may bring the patient directly into X-ray."

Before the waiting room of patients had time to figure out why a woman with a cat carrier was in an internist's office, she had disappeared into the inner offices.

The X-ray technician was ready. While the woman soothed her cat, the technician placed the X-ray cone over the cat's leg and held her securely with a lead glove.

The cat and its owner waited for the technician to develop the film. When it was ready, Dr. Prutting was called in. He looked at the X-ray and said he thought the leg looked pretty good but was not completely healed, and that the wire should stay in place a little longer. The only trouble was how much longer. That was one answer Dr. Prutting couldn't come up with.

By sheer coincidence I showed up at the office at that moment. I had just a minor ache but I was concerned, and I was aware that I hadn't seen Dr. Prutting in a year. Because I couldn't be sure when my own schedule would allow me to get away, I hadn't made an appointment; I just waited until I was in the neighborhood. I expected a long wait, especially when I saw the place filled with patients, so I was amazed when the nurse immediately ushered me back to the office area. "I know Dr. Prutting will want to see you right away."

What did that mean? Did she know something about my health that I didn't know? I was more surprised when she took me to the X-ray room.

Dr. Prutting looked up as I entered, and he was even more surprised than I was.

He handed the X-ray to me, and I corroborated his diagnosis. I said to the woman, "Take the cat and this X-ray back to the animal hospital in three weeks. I think they'll agree the wire can come out then."

The next day, I sent a large package by messenger to Dr. Prutting's office.

He was still laughing when he telephoned to thank me. I had sent him *Merck's Manual of Veterinary Medicine* with a note attached: "If you're going to do it, you may as well do it right."

Chapter 12

I DON'T SEE too many kittens being born. Considering how long I've been a veterinarian involved with the cat population of New York City, it may seem surprising when I say that. Perhaps it's because I won't do breeder work. I urge all my clients to have their animals neutered to keep down the unwanted-pet population, and, as cats are marvelous mothers, I get calls from clients only when the mother-to-be is in trouble. And, of course, since mine is largely an apartment-cat practice, my female patients don't have many opportunities to get in the family way, as we used to say. Without a male in residence, just how is it going to happen?

But happen it does. An occasional backyard foray, a window-sill tête-a-tête, or a little get-together that occurred before the cat became a client's pet can result in an unexpected litter. I usually find out about the coming blessed event when a client calls, not knowing the cat is pregnant, to ask what to feed his overweight animal or to question her strange new habit of hiding.

A cat who is about to deliver gets very definite ideas about where she wants to give birth. It's not that she's trying to keep her babies to herself, it's that she is trying to protect them. Her instincts tell her to find a place where her kittens will be safe from predators. Granted, there may not be any predators in the apartment, but that has nothing to do with the instincts guiding the mother cat.

The place she chooses will be an out-of-the-way, usually dark, corner. And it is a place she must select herself. To try to select a place for your cat is a waste of time as far as the cat and I are concerned. She probably will not use it. If at all possible, let the cat make her choice, and put up with it. Quite often it will be her usual hiding place—in a closet or under a bed. Of course, if she decides the perfect place to have her litter is the front hall, blocking the door to the apartment, then you have to help her find something better from your point of view.

I once received a frantic late-night call from a very upset lady. "My cat is having kittens right on my bed—between my legs! What should I do?"

"Not a damn thing," I said. "She obviously thinks that's the ideal place. Wait until she's all done, then get up and make her a bed of towels or of a blanket you don't need. Put her on the floor on top of it with her kittens, and then go back to sleep."

The lady sounded most unhappy with my advice. "But what about all the blood?"

"She'll clean up as much as she can. You'll have to explain the rest as best you can to your laundry."

I didn't know why the woman didn't sound more pleased at her cat's choice of place to give birth. She should have been honored. Actress-dancer Beverley Bozeman Fuller certainly was when Pansy gave birth to her first litter in Mrs. Fuller's lap. It was when Pansy tried to do it again (the first litter had ruined Beverley's best slacks) that she drew the line. Mrs. Fuller called to her family to bring towels and she gently lifted Pansy off her lap and set her into them. Pansy made it clear that she wanted Beverley, her husband, Dean, and young John and Liza Fuller with her during the whole procedure, and they were happy to oblige. All of which makes Pansy an unusual cat, since most cats normally prefer privacy when giving birth.

Martini, the Siamese belonging to Frances and Richard Lock-ridge, did all the right things as her perfectly normal nine-week pregnancy was coming to an end. She made her nest in the back of a closet and went into what seemed like normal labor while the Lockridges kept an eye on her from a distance. But after she had been in her hideaway for nine or ten hours and no kitten was forthcoming, they telephoned me.

I told them they were right to call. That was too long for labor to continue unassisted. Obviously, Martini needed help. I told the Lockridges to cover the kitchen table with clean sheets or towels they didn't care about, and to move Martini there for me. After what the cat had been going through in her own place, I doubted that she'd fight the move. She didn't.

I rushed right over and examined Martini to determine the cause of the dystocia. Maternal dystocia means a pelvic abnormality or blockage or other problem with the mother. Fetal dystocia means the problem is with the kitten. I couldn't determine which it was.

Since the poor Siamese had been in labor so long, I knew the uterine muscles were getting lax from all those contractions. So I gave her a shot of Pituitrin to encourage her hormone activity and assist the muscle tone for continuing labor.

Soon the shot had its effect, and as Martini pushed, I massaged her belly along with her contractions. Between the two of us, Martini and I got the first kitten down the uterine tubes and out.

I'd better stop and explain that. While a tubular pregnancy is an abnormality in a human being, cats and all multiparates—animals that normally give birth to more than one at a time—have what you might call tubular pregnancies. In multiparates the womb is shaped like an upside-down V. The two tubes are actually part of the uterus, which is where the fertilized egg stays and develops.

In the early stages of a cat's pregnancy—the third to the fifth week—a trained hand can feel the pea-sized lumps that are the kittens in the two tubes and know how many kittens there will be. Towards the end of pregnancy—the point at which Martini was—it is impossible to feel the separate bodies because they move together.

142

Since I had not done an early pregnancy examination on Martini, I didn't have the foggiest idea how many kittens were to follow the first. After cutting the umbilical cord and giving Martini the placenta to eat, activating the hormones to help the mother produce milk for her kittens, I rubbed the first kitten to get its circulation going and clean it a bit and gave it to Martini.

Normally, cats purr straight through the delivery of their litters. But not Martini. The poor thing had been through so much pain for such a long time, she took it out on Richard Lockridge, biting the hell out of his hands as he held her on the table.

After a little rest, I gave her another shot of Pituitrin. She squeezed and squeezed, and the back end of a second kitten appeared. With firm, positive, but gentle tugs, I helped the kitten out. There were only two in her litter.

Martini was still not purring, but at last she relaxed. We put her back in her chosen place with her kittens beside her. To look at the three of them, you would have thought it was the easiest birth in the world.

Before I left, the Lockridges asked about the sex of the kittens. "One boy, one girl," I said, put on my hat and left. A few months later, when it was time to neuter the kittens, named Gin and Sherry, I had to confess to the Lockridges that I had made a mistake. Both kittens were females. "Listen," I said sheepishly, "at the beginning it's hard to tell—even for a vet."

I wouldn't swear that the Lockridges held my mistake against me, but I do know they portrayed me rather shabbily in one of their many Mr. and Mrs. North mysteries, *The Judge Is Reversed.* Though the character was named Dr. Oscar Gebhardt, I knew it had to be me. How many balding cat doctors did they know with an office on Park Avenue who prefer to make house calls? They even sneaked a case of difficult parturition on 10th Street, their block, into the story.

Several years later, after Frances died, Richard wrote a charming book called *One Lady, Two Cats* about the introduction of his new wife, Hildy, to Martini's successors, Pammy and Sherry (the second). Richard treated me a lot more kindly in that book, but then he had to—that one is nonfiction.

Thinking of kittens makes me think of babies, and that makes me think of an old wives' tale that it's time to get rid of. Believe it or not, just when I think I've heard the last of this bit of nonsense, someone asks me if it's true that cats can hurt a baby by sucking its breath. Absolute sheer and utter nonsense.

A cat may leap up on the crib to take a look at the new baby when it comes home from the hospital, but that's mere curiosity, not a desire to suck its breath. Cats live on meat, not babies' breath. Once the cat has satisfied its curiosity as to what the new thing is in the house, it usually decides that the baby is of no interest, and goes on about its own business.

Watching your cat—or helping her, if she will allow it—bring her kittens into the world can be unforgettable.

My own doctor, John Prutting, and his family were eagerly looking forward to their cat's imminent motherhood. The Pruttings agreed that it would be a good learning experience for their young daughter.

Since their two gray tabbies had been born backstage during the initial Broadway run of the musical *Finian's Rainbow,* they were named for two of the leading characters in the show, Sharon and Woody.

The afternoon that Sharon went into labor the three Pruttings gathered to watch. What was expected to be a beautiful experience turned into a sad one when Sharon, with great difficulty, delivered herself of three stillborn kittens. The Pruttings consoled their daughter as best they could.

But that evening, Jane Prutting came running into her husband's study to tell him that Sharon was about to have another kitten. "Come quickly, John. This looks like it's going to be a fine one."

Again the three Pruttings gathered in the kitchen near the corner by the stove that Sharon had chosen. John was nervous

144

about the new kitten's coming, partly for Sharon and partly for his daughter. "Get Camuti!" he shouted to no one in particular.

Jane Prutting telephoned me and I said I'd get there as quickly as I could.

John Prutting got a warm cloth and watched Sharon's progress, easing her kitten into the world as gently as he'd learned to do with human deliveries. Though he acted calmly and professionally with Sharon, he kept fretting to his wife, daughter, even Woody, "Where's Camuti? Why doesn't he get here?" Later he admitted he had acted just the way his own patients' hysterical families behaved.

Sharon's kitten took only five minutes to be born, alive and healthy. The mother ate the placenta, licked her baby clean and curled up with it.

Then something happened that I wish I had been there to see. It took everyone by surprise.

Woody, the kitten's father, came over to the box in which Sharon lay with her baby. A large and husky cat, Woody, very gently and without extruding any claws, reached into the basket and touched the tiny newborn kitten. It was a very light, delicate pat.

Then, in slow motion, he withdrew his paw and slowly backed away. As the Pruttings watched in astonishment, Woody went over to a toy dog he sometimes played with, picked it up in his mouth and carried it to his sleeping basket, which was near Sharon's box. He hopped into his basket and curled up with the toy just as Sharon was doing with her kitten.

When I arrived, the three Pruttings took me into the kitchen. John put a finger to his lips to tell me to be very quiet. I looked from Sharon in her box to Woody in his basket. Each was curled up and asleep with its "child."

I saw that everything was all right, and I left.

Chapter 13

I CAN'T SAY I'm overly impressed by celebrities or millionaires. Cats are my business, and they come with the people who take care of them. Some of those people have been celebrities. But the only thing that impresses me is how well the owner takes care of his or her pet, not how famous the owner is. There have even been times when I've had to be told who the owner was because I didn't recognize him. When you have a nighttime practice, you don't go to the theater very often or to many movies, so I've never been up on who the big names are. And by the time I sit down in front of my television set to relax before going to bed, the only stars I see are people like Randolph Scott and Irene Dunne.

But there have been some people I've liked who also happened to be celebrities. Imogene Coca was one, also James and Pamela Mason. As for Tallulah Bankhead, I can't say that I actually liked her. But I certainly remember her.

It was the comedienne Jane Dulo, a client of mine, who recommended me to Miss Coca. At the time I met her she was just becoming a household word as the costar with Sid Caesar on the Saturday night television program "Your Show of Shows." She lived with her mother, Sadie, and her cat, Gainzer, in a Beekman Place apartment.

The building was delighted with Imogene Coca and her

mother, but Gainzer was continuously in trouble. It was the man in the adjoining penthouse who blew the whistle on Gainzer and went charging in on Sadie to raise hell about the cat, whom he had caught rooting around in his well-tended garden. Not only had Gainzer torn up some of his plants, but she had added insult to injury by using the man's planters for litter boxes.

Sadie apologized and promised to confine Gainzer to the apartment, which turned out to be easier said than done. When Gainzer discovered she could no longer go out the terrace door, she made the front door her exit. Gainzer took to lurking around the front door waiting for it to open. The minute guests or a delivery man came to the door, Gainzer shot down the hall to the service stairs. The whole building became her stalking ground, and search parties were frequently organized to find her. Mrs. Coca would call down to the doorman whenever the cat disappeared, and he in turn would alert the elevator operators. The entire building staff had orders to stop Gainzer on sight. Gainzer was usually returned in a very short time.

Gainzer was one of the few longhairs I've known who didn't wash herself well and frequently suffered from matted fur, no matter how often and carefully she was brushed. The summer after the Cocas moved to Beekman Place, it happened again.

Because her matted fur caused a skin irritation, Gainzer became sulky and subdued. The only advantage to her discomfort was that it kept Gainzer housebound. But finally, Sadie Coca called me to give Gainzer one of "those haircuts," as she called them.

What I did was shave Gainzer completely except for a ruff of fur around the head, and a little clump at the tip of the tail. Those were the two areas unaffected by Gainzer's rash, which I treated with ointment. To give Gainzer her due, she never seemed to mind her haircuts.

Shortly after the trimming session, with the ointment relieving her discomfort, Gainzer's passion for travel resumed.

As soon as she missed the cat, Mrs. Coca started her usual series of calls, alerting the doorman and the elevator staff before she headed down the service stairs where she occasionally trapped Gainzer. But this time she found nothing.

Mrs. Coca returned to her apartment and telephoned all of the people with penthouse terraces. None of them had seen the cat. Mrs. Coca went out again and spoke personally to the elevator men and the doorman, the superintendent, the handyman and the porters. She told the entire building staff that she would pay a reward to the man who brought Gainzer back. The doorman, doing his best to gear up for the hunt, slipped away from his post and went to the supply closet where he kept a bottle. On his next break, the doorman went back to the supply room. By the time he came out he was weaving, but he began his hunt, anxious to get the reward money, which would help him to keep his supply room stocked.

Mrs. Coca was startled when she opened the door and heard the doorman say, "I'm sorry to tell you this but your cat has been eaten."

Horrified, Mrs. Coca demanded more information.

"Well, I can't be sure but I'll bet I know what's happened. There's a wild lion downstairs and he must have eaten the cat."

Mrs. Coca asked to be taken to the landing on the service stairs where the doorman had sighted the lion. She found Gainzer, hiding behind an empty garbage pail. When Mrs. Coca called to tell me the story, she said, "Gainzer did look a little like a lion. I just hope she doesn't take this new role seriously."

Tallulah Bankhead may have been a great actress, but she could also be a great nuisance and a spoiled child. Despite it all, she was warm and touching, when you didn't want to strangle her. I met her first in the 1950's through the well-known jazz pianist, Joe Bushkin, who had given her a Maltese pup from his dog's litter. She had named her Maltese Delores for Burr Tilstrom's puppet, and called me to check it out.

When I arrived at the Elysée where she was staying, there was the great Tallulah, looking pretty much the way she did in pictures I had seen of her. She was slim, wearing slacks and sweater, her hair a loose mane around her head. In one hand she held a drink, in the other a cigarette. When she said hello, the voice was the famous Bankhead baritone.

She was alone, a rare occurrence that I didn't appreciate because it was my first visit. Only in later visits did I realize that wherever Tallulah was, there was always a mob in residence.

I looked around for Delores but didn't see her. Miss Bankhead said, "How about a drink?"

"I don't drink," I said, waiting to get on with the business I had come for. I saw the Bankhead eyebrows lift as she tried to figure out what was wrong with me that I didn't drink.

"Where's the dog?"

Tallulah waved a hand loosely around the apartment. "Delores will show up any minute now."

She sat down on the couch, put her feet up on the coffee table and indicated that I was to sit in the chair opposite so we could talk a bit about Delores.

I noticed as I turned to sit down that there was a tall piece of furniture behind me. The minute I sat down, I heard a voice from behind me say, "It's time to go home."

It startled me, but when I looked around I couldn't see anyone. Miss Bankhead, who was a nonstop talker went right on with whatever she was saying.

A few minutes later, that voice came again. "What's your telephone number?"

Tallulah caught that. "Don't pay any attention to Chico," she said. "He's a mynah bird."

Finally Delores appeared, and I examined her. The animal was healthy. While I was there, something dropped on my shoulder. I figured it was a piece of loose plaster from the ceiling and went about my business.

When I got to my next house call, the client helped me off with my coat and said, "Dr. Camuti, were you walking in the park without your overcoat at this time of the year?"

"What are you talking about?" I said to the woman.

149

She pointed to my jacket. "There's bird dirt on your shoulder."

I thought of the Bankhead kitchen. The next time I went to see Delores I told Miss Bankhead what had happened. She wasn't the least bit embarrassed. "That's Gaylord, shame on him."

Gaylord turned out to be a parakeet that had the complete run of the Bankhead apartment. She didn't bother to keep him caged. When I said I didn't like it, she promised to put Gaylord in his cage whenever I came.

With each visit I seemed to discover another resident of the Bankhead apartment. There was Chico the mynah bird; Gaylord the parakeet; Delores the Maltese; Dolly, a Siamese cat who for some unknown reason spent most of the time with Irving Hoffman, the columnist; and a Pekingese named Gabrielle.

At the time that Gabrielle had to be spayed, Tallulah Bankhead was preparing to appear in a production of *A Streetcar Named Desire*. I performed Gabrielle's surgery at my office and then sent her back to the Elysée.

The time for Gabrielle's stitches to come out was the day before Tallulah was leaving for Key West to go over the play with Tennessee Williams. I telephoned and told her the stitches had to come out before she left town. "Are you taking the dogs with you?" I asked.

"Of course, and we leave tomorrow morning."

"Then the stitches have to come out this afternoon."

It turned out that she would not be home. I told her to have someone at the apartment to let me in and I'd stop by and remove the stitches.

She agreed, but when I went by the Elysée later that afternoon, I was told there was no one in the Bankhead apartment. I asked for the hotel manager and explained about Gabrielle's stitches.

He shook his head. "I'm sorry, but I just can't let you in there."

We argued back and forth. Finally, I said, "Look, I'm going to need some help, anyway. Why don't you send someone from your staff along with me? That way you don't have to worry about anything going wrong in the apartment."

The bell captain went with me and held Delores while I removed her stitches. It had taken longer to get into the apartment than it had to remove the stitches. By the time I finished I was steaming mad at Tallulah Bankhead for not remembering to have someone at the apartment to let me in. I decided to write her a stinging note. I reached for what I at first thought was a notebook and tore a page out of it. It was then that I saw the printing on the page and realized it was part of the acting script of *A Streetcar Named Desire*. But I was too angry to care. I turned the page over and ripped into Miss Bankhead for wasting so much of my time. Stars!

To this day I don't know whether or not Tallulah Bankhead ever missed that page of dialogue. For all I know she went through the run of her show making a one-page leap at every performance.

In time my anger passed. It was difficult to stay angry with Tallulah Bankhead, and she certainly couldn't be faulted as a pet owner. For all the nuisance she sometimes was, she still fulfilled all my requirements. She paid her bills, she followed my instructions for her animals, and she seemed to care about them very much.

One night I went up to see Delores and found Tallulah, as usual, in the midst of a bunch of friends. Why she had them there I can't imagine, since she couldn't speak. She had laryngitis. She wrote me a note to say Delores was in the kitchen and that a nose-and-throat specialist was coming to see about the laryngitis.

While I was checking Delores in the kitchen, Tallulah's doctor arrived. He was a short, shy man—made twice as shy by the freeloaders in the living room, all of whom ignored him—and he was dressed in evening clothes. He explained that he was on the way to the opera but didn't want to keep Miss Bankhead waiting until morning.

The doctor, flustered by the mob in the living room, suggested that Miss Bankhead take him to her bedroom for the examination. I was just coming from the kitchen as the doctor and Tallulah came out of the bedroom. She walked him to the front door where he stopped and turned beet red. He realized that he had forgotten to give her a shot of antibiotics.

Tallulah nodded, lifted up her dress in front of everyone in the room, and bent over the sofa. "Okay," she croaked, "give it to me here."

She wasn't wearing panties and the poor doctor nearly died of embarrassment. For that matter, so did I.

"Would you mind going back into the bedroom?" he said.

Tallulah shrugged, dropped her dress and went off to the bedroom again. No one in the living room seemed fazed by the incident, but her two doctors were completely rattled.

I once asked her, "Why do you have all these parasites around, eating your food, drinking your liquor?"

"I always have to have people around me," she said. "Even when I go to the bathroom I want somebody with me to hold my hand."

She didn't say that to shock me though I was startled at the time. It was just Tallulah speaking the truth about herself. Despite all the noise and the mob that always surrounded her, you could sense a loneliness that she never seemed to defeat.

Tallulah Bankhead rarely if ever did anything quietly and without fuss, and traveling was no exception. She called one day to tell me she was planning a trip to California. She was certain that all of her friends out there wanted to meet Dolly and Delores.

"That's crazy," I said. "Take Delores with you if you want, but leave Dolly home. Everyone knows what a cat looks like, even in California. And she'll be much happier at home."

The Bankhead voice grew icy with dignity. "I'm not calling to ask you, I'm calling to tell you I'm taking them." And she hung up on me.

Fifteen minutes later she called again. "You had nothing to do with it. It wasn't what you said to me, but I, myself, have decided to take Delores on the trip and leave Dolly with Irving Hoffman."

"Okay," I said.

"But I'm taking United's night plane so I think I should have something to sedate Delores."

That made sense to me. In those days the night planes were Boeing 247's and had sleeping berths. The trip took about seventeen hours.

I gave her some phenobarbital tablets, and advised one for each flight.

Unfortunately, the suggested dosage wasn't strong enough. Halfway across country Delores woke up and started barking, waking up everyone in the neighboring berths.

Tallulah called me from California to tell me about the flight. I told her that for the return trip Delores would require a stronger dosage, and I added that I was certain she could find all the pills she needed in Beverly Hills. Miss Bankhead balked. She wanted me to send her the pills.

"I'm not going to mail pills across the country," I said. I took the telephone away from my ear, knowing what would happen next.

Sure enough, there was a sharp click as Tallulah hung up on me. Since I was getting used to that treatment I stayed near the telephone, waiting for the next call.

A few minutes later the phone rang again. "Are you going to send me that medicine?"

"No," I said. She hung up on me again.

Ten minutes later, the third call came. "I'll have somebody stop by and pick it up."

One time, she called to announce that she was going to appear at the Sands in Las Vegas and she was taking Delores with her. I suggested that if she liked I could give Delores a shot for the trip. She liked the idea and asked me to meet her at her place and go with her to La Guardia.

A chauffeured limousine drove us out. One of her many stooges sat up front beside the chauffeur holding Delores. Tallulah and I sat in the back. She was in slacks and was clutching an enormous bag crammed with makeup and assorted pills. Every two minutes she'd stick her head up front to ask the driver, "How soon do we get there?"

"We're way ahead of time," I said. "You won't miss your plane."

"You don't understand," she said impatiently. "When a celebrity arrives there are always reporters and photographers waiting. I want to get myself ready."

With that she turned the bag upside down and dumped everything onto the car floor. She began poking around to find the right lipstick, rouge, a comb, and so on.

When we arrived at United Airlines at La Guardia, there wasn't a single reporter or photographer on hand to greet her. Tallulah looked at me. "Do you think some other celebrity is here?"

If there were any reporters or photographers around La Guardia who didn't know that the great Tallulah had arrived, they soon found out as her luggage started being unloaded—she had enough to fill a plane all by herself—and her entourage closed in on us. There was the guy who had been holding Delores; her lawyer; hairdresser; manicurist; secretary; three or four friends; her maid, Rose; and believe it or not, her dentist. You could hear the racket clear to Manhattan as the small army, which now included several redcaps, moved toward the United desk. Tallulah's voice dominated everything.

The agent immediately spotted Delores's carrier. "What's that?"

"That's for my dog," Tallulah said.

"Oh, you can't use that. The dog must go in an airline carrier."

"Don't be silly, young man," Tallulah said in her most imperious voice. "Delores will travel in her own carrier."

By now, most of the other travelers and bystanders within a mile knew that a VIP was there, and a crowd gathered. The Bankhead baritone rode above everything as she told the clerk in no uncertain terms that his rules were petty and she couldn't be bothered even listening to them.

Somebody called the manager, who came over and repeated everything the clerk had said, and then Tallulah told him everything she had said to the clerk. The manager looked like a reasonable man to me, so I convinced Tallulah I could handle everything. I sent her and her assorted chums and entourage off to the VIP Lounge. Most of the crowd of onlookers followed her.

"Look," I said to the manager, "let her carry the dog on the plane in her own carrier. When she's on board, you can have the stewardess bring her the airline carrier. With no crowd around to play to, I think she'll go along with you people."

"Fine," he said. I didn't bother to explain that the dog was going to be anesthetized and wouldn't need any carrier.

Tallulah, Delores, and I boarded the plane before the other passengers. It was one of the new DC-7s with a circular lounge at the back. Tallulah put Delores on one of the lounge tables and I gave her the shot. The dog was asleep in minutes.

Tallulah carried Delores up front to the bulkhead seat and put her on the floor at her feet. We told the stewardess about the anesthesia and that Miss Bankhead would have to turn the dog every hour to keep its lungs from becoming congested. All things considered, there was no need for a carrier. The stewardess agreed.

I said goodbye to Miss Bankhead and left the plane. I thought that was the end of the whole crazy business. Suddenly, there was shouting behind me, and there was Tallulah Bankhead and the stewardess at the top of the stairs, waving and yelling. I went back. "Now what?"

"The dog is dead," Tallulah said.

"Nonsense," I said.

"Come see for yourself!"

I entered the plane and knelt beside Delores for a minute. "The dog is perfectly fine," I said, tipped my hat and left again.

The minute I got to the limousine I barked at the chauffeur, "Let's get out of here fast before that loony starts calling me again!"

Needless to say, everything went just fine on the flight. Delores slept all the way to Las Vegas, which I could have predicted. And Tallulah turned the dog every hour, which I could also have predicted.

She may have acted high-handedly and even indifferently with people, but when it came to her pets Tallulah gave them better care than she took of even herself.

I could never say that Tallulah Bankhead was an easy person to be around. To spend time with her was like hanging around with a hurricane. You never knew what would happen or how severe the storm would be from one minute to the next. But I can look back on her in memory and smile. There was love in the woman, and it came out in her treatment of her pets.

I don't know why it is that people think actors are just like the people they play. Why should the man who makes his living making people laugh be funny at home? Or why should we think that a woman who plays sexy tramps in the movies is a sexy tramp in real life? If that were the case, they wouldn't be actors.

Of the actors I've gotten to know through my work, very few of them were like the people they played on the stage or screen. James Mason is a good example of what I mean. When you think of him, what probably comes to mind is the very smooth, polished type who turns out to be an enemy agent or a murderer. As the veterinarian who took care of his cats for awhile, when I think of him I remember one of the most warm-hearted and concerned cat lovers I have ever known.

To tell you about James Mason and his wife at the time, Pamela Kellino, I have to begin with Hattie Gray Baker, who recommended me to them.

Miss Baker worked as a movie censor in the New York office of Twentieth Century-Fox. It was her job to read new scripts before they were filmed and to tell the writers what wouldn't get through the censorship code that existed at that time. She also checked on the films as the shooting progressed. It was the private screenings of the completed films—together with Miss

Baker's love for her cats—that nearly cost her her job several times.

Twentieth Century-Fox had its screening room—a private movie theater—in its West Side offices. When a film was completed, it would be shown for the top executives and Hattie. Because Hattie loved her cats so much, and because she had seen the films in bits and pieces so many times during their making, she often forgot herself during the final screenings.

The picture would have just begun and the executive next to her would have settled back in his seat to study the product when Hattie would lean toward him and say, "Did I tell you what my cat did last night?"

The executive often bounded out of his seat and signaled to the projectionist to stop the film, rewind it and start the screening all over again. Hattie's face would grow red, and she would slink down in her seat, feeling about two inches tall.

"I sure loused up many an afternoon talking about my cats," Hattie told me. But she must have been good at her job because she was never fired.

I met James and Pamela Mason in 1947 when they first came to New York from England to star in a play called *Bathsheba,* which was not a great success. Never a one-cat family, they arrived in America with five cats and a dog, as well as a staff to take care of the Masons and their pets. The Masons divided their time between a rented house in Greenwich, Connecticut, and an apartment in New York City. They spent Monday, Tuesday, Thursday and Friday nights in New York, and the other nights, as well as all day Sunday, in Connecticut.

The cats did not have to commute. They stayed at the house in Greenwich. Unfortunately the staff couldn't keep an eye on all the cats who went in and out of the house, a habit they had picked up at their English country home. One day, Tree, a favorite Siamese, disappeared.

The Masons went wild with worry. They took out ads in all the local papers. They contacted the local ASPCA, put up notices around the neighborhood, called all the veterinarians for miles around, talked to neighbors and especially local children. They called the police and hired private detectives to search for Tree, and they offered a reward for the cat's return. They even wired Louella Parsons, the Hollywood columnist, to make an appeal for Tree's return over her radio show. When the Masons were in New York appearing in their play, Violet, their housekeeper, kept up the search, walking through the woods late into the night calling for Tree. As you can see, James Mason's behavior was hardly that of a movie villain.

Naturally, people started telephoning the Masons, and they followed up on every call. But none of them led to Tree.

Six days after Tree disappeared Violet called the Masons in New York City to tell them that two men had brought home Tree's body. Tragically, the Siamese had been found dead on the side of the Merritt Parkway, several miles from the house.

The Masons rushed up to Greenwich and took Tree's body to the local vet. They assumed that Tree had died of exhaustion, but they wanted to know for certain. The veterinarian told them that Tree had been killed by an automobile. But, the doctor said, Tree couldn't have walked all those miles to the spot where his body was found without showing signs of such a journey on his paws. It was obvious that Tree had been catnapped.

Since Tree had never been a wanderer, just a garden-sitter, the criminal or criminals must have picked the cat right out of the Masons' yard, and then for some unknown reason let him go. The poor thing never had a chance of getting home. After twelve years of adoration for that cat, the Masons, like all other cat lovers, took his death very hard.

Losing Tree soured the Masons on Greenwich and shortly afterward they moved their country residence to Riverdale, New York, where I met them. At first they didn't talk much about Tree. His death was too painful to them.

But with the passage of time, they began to tell me about him. He was a shy and gentle creature who didn't take to new people in his life too easily. But the Masons remembered with laughter one English neighbor in Beaconsfield who became Tree's friend. Tree met her by following the afternoon sun to her garden. The meeting was obviously a pleasant one for Tree and he took to dropping in on her several times a week. And then one day, Tree returned home with a souvenir of his afternoon's visit—an entire roast chicken!

The ground was muddy that day, but Tree was a very neat and gentlemanly Siamese. He held the chicken high above the ground, so that it arrived home in perfect condition except for one set of teeth marks.

Tree was obviously very proud of himself as he laid his catch at the feet of his owners. The Masons made a big fuss over his prowess, even as they worried about what to do with the "hot chicken," as they called it. They had a hunch that the neighbor might not understand, and they didn't want to cool her devotion to Tree.

There was only one solution that they could come up with. They served a chicken dinner to Tree, Topboy, Nibbler (who belonged to Violet), Whitey and Lady Leeds—all the cats in the Mason household—and kept the drumsticks for themselves.

In time, James Mason's career took him, Pamela and their cats to California. One day I got a letter from Pamela telling me that they were expecting a child. But, she joked, "I'd rather have a Burmese kitten."

When their daughter, Portland, was born, I sent them a telegram: "Don't forget the distemper shots!"

In 1949, James and Pamela Mason published a book, *The Cats in Our Lives,* a warm and delightful memoir of their four-footed friends. I especially like their explanation of what it is about cats that make some people love them and others detest them:

Dogs as a general rule tend to keep asking one, "What would you advise me to do now? I just sit doing nothing. There must be something that would give me fun. Why don't you start something for me? You're a man; you must know better than I what I want to do."

I don't happen to be equipped with the will to influence people. Therefore I disappoint dogs, much as I like them, for they all but insist on being influenced.

I do not think I disappoint cats. Whether they like it or not, I influence them to the extent of encouraging good manners. They do not need to be shown how to have a good time, for they are unfailingly ingenious in that respect. Nor do they need to be told who is the master, for it is a matter of extreme indifference to them. They are affectionate to those whom they recognize as friends and humor them by falling in with their wishes, provided they are not too whimsical.

When those who do not know cats find themselves in a house which is given over to them, they generally want to have the thing explained. In many families the superiority of dog is a tradition so firmly established that their members find it hard to accept the idea that some people prefer cats. Never having enjoyed a friendly relationship with cats, they cannot imagine what the fuss is all about. Ten to one they falsely conclude that cat lovers are automatically dog haters. Cat lovers are so used to this that most of them have their own prepared statements on the subject, beginning with the words: "It's not that we dislike dogs. It's just that we like cats better. . . ." *

I guess that of all my celebrity encounters, my favorite story —and it's a joke on me—concerns the celebrity I didn't even notice.

The woman wasn't my client, but the mother of my client. Whenever I went to see the daughter's Siamese, there was the mother butting in to ask me a thousand questions. I liked the daughter but I hated going to the house because of her mother.

Then the Siamese had kittens and they developed ringworm, which meant several visits. I don't think there was one time that

* *The Cats in Our Lives* by Pamela Kellino and James Mason. Illustrated by James Mason. Current Books, Inc., A.A. Wyn, Publisher, New York, 1949.

I showed up at the house without that mother being there, firing questions at me. Why did I do this? What caused that? I couldn't work for the interruptions.

Finally, after one such visit I took my client aside as I was leaving. "Look, I like you very much," I said, "and I think you are pleased with me. But I can't take your mother and all those questions any more. Keep her out of the room. Tell her I can't stop everything to talk to her. Or better yet, find some excuse so she won't be here at all!"

I'd always leave the apartment fuming, and Alex would have to try to calm me down before we arrived at the next stop.

One evening, we were home watching television. Alex was in the kitchen doing something when suddenly I saw the daughter on the television screen. "Alex!" I shouted, "come here quick. It's Mrs. Riva, the one with the mother!"

Alex came running. She took one look at the daughter, whose name was Maria Riva—Mrs. William Riva was all I ever knew—and said, "Don't you realize who that is?"

"Yeah, the girl with the pesty mother," I said.

Alex shook her head in disbelief. "Lou, that's Marlene Dietrich's daughter! The woman who was bothering you was Marlene Dietrich!"

"Well, I just thought she was a pain in the neck."

Alex got that look of long-term suffering she sometimes uses on me. "Didn't you notice her legs?"

"Why should I? I was there to look at ringworm."

Another type of celebrity I've come across through my medical practice is the millionaire. Truth to tell, I don't really consider millionaires celebrities. I think money's a pretty nice thing to have, but it's nothing much to be celebrated for.

While I've met some charming and happy millionaires, I think they were the exception to the rule. And the happy ones, as I remember them, were the ones who *made* the fortunes, not the ones who inherited them.

You can have most of the millionaires who were my clients.

Most of them left me feeling uneasy and depressed. I suppose if I ever needed proof that money can't buy happiness I learned it from them. But then again, as someone once said, maybe money can't buy happiness but it can make unhappiness a lot more pleasant.

I can't particularly say that Doris Duke left me with a happy feeling, but she was a nice lady. Her father started the American Tobacco Company. He became so wealthy and gave so much money to a North Carolina college that they changed the school's name to Duke University. Doris Duke was thirteen years old when her father died, and she inherited more than $70,000,000.

I met Miss Duke in 1936 shortly after her marriage to James Cromwell. Now, what does a man give his bride when she already has millions? James Cromwell presented Doris Duke Cromwell with two Siamese cats. Enter Camuti.

She asked me down to her country place, Duke Farms, in Somerville, New Jersey, to check over her new Siamese. She was an attractive, slim young lady dressed in dungarees when she greeted me. Now, the Camutis may have carried the title of count in the old country and lived a comfortable life, but it couldn't compare to Duke Farms. I have had a good enough upbringing not to be overly impressed by wealth, but it wasn't good enough to make me ignore a 2,000-acre estate with 125 in staff. And on the way to the main house, Doris Duke took me through the greenhouse, where she grew orchids by the thousands.

After we had sat a while, she with her legs tossed over the arm of a chair, and talked about the cats and how she should be taking care of them, she asked if I would like to see the estate. I leaped at the chance and she ordered a car brought around. It turned out to be a seven-seat open touring car.

She got behind the wheel and I sat beside her. "There's just one thing I want to tell you," she said. "The dogs may resent it if you get too close to me or touch me. If you keep that in mind everything will be fine."

With that she called out, and three of the biggest Great Danes I'd ever seen came bounding across the lawn and leaped up into the back seat of the car. I froze. Just the thought that if I made a move they didn't like they might rip me apart made me break out in a cold sweat. Yet I was too paralyzed to reach for a handkerchief to wipe my brow.

Doris Duke started the motor and we were off on what seemed like the longest trip of my life, though it took actually under an hour. Throughout the entire tour the dogs kept licking the back of my balding head and covering my scalp with warm, sticky saliva. I was fit to be tied, but I still didn't move. Miss Duke didn't seem to notice what was going on, and she kept rattling away about this or that building on her property while I sat there, stiff as a flagpole, feeling stinking wet and slimy.

Finally the grand tour ended. As soon as we got back to the house I had to strip to the waist to clean myself. I hadn't thought Doris Duke was aware of the washing her dogs had given me, but there was a knock at the bathroom door and it was her hand that came in holding a large bath towel for me.

I paid professional visits to the then Mrs. Cromwell several times at her country place and also in the city at the big house at 78th and Fifth Avenue where her mother lived. Not that I saw much of Doris Duke. Usually it was just a servant who took me to the two Siamese. I would treat them for whatever was the matter, mail in my bill and get paid by the estate. Everything was handled in a businesslike way until the new husband got into the act.

It all began with Pete, one of the two Siamese who was having some sort of problem which required my X-raying him in the city, and then seeing him several times after he had been taken out to Duke Farms. I suggested that Mrs. Cromwell find a local veterinarian out there, but she said she wanted me.

I went, and when the series of treatments was completed I sent in my bill. I received a very curt letter from Elizabeth Knox, a secretary, who accused me of billing Mrs. Cromwell exorbitantly at the rate of $385 for seven house calls and the New York City X-ray.

While I'd have to agree that the charge was steep, it took me a whole day to go to and from Somerville, which meant that I couldn't see any other clients that day. If Mrs. Cromwell wanted me, I didn't see why I should lose money on the deal.

Miss Knox further raised my hackles in her letter by telling me about an osteopath who came from Philadelphia to the farm to treat Mr. *and* Mrs. Cromwell for an hour and a half and only charged $25 for his visit.

I wrote to Miss Knox that I was sorry about the situation but neither she nor Mrs. Cromwell had asked me about my fee in advance of my visits, and that I couldn't be expected to place a value on my time as another doctor might his. The least I would accept was $15 per hour or $75 per call.

A week later I received a letter from Cromwell himself, a letter which held little charm. Among other things he said, "I am writing to ask you not to make any further visits as I consider your charges for such service beyond all reason, in fact, I consider them preposterous under the circumstances."

Exasperated, I sat down at my typewriter and wrote him to just send a check for whatever amount he wanted, and be done with it. I didn't need such letters.

Naturally, I got another letter from him, a long one, telling me the osteopath story all over again, and adding that the osteopath had an even greater distance to drive than I did. Therefore, Mr. Cromwell wrote, I would be paid the same $25 per visit as the osteopath plus $10 for the City visit. He enclosed a check for $285.

I wrote back to him that it would be my pleasure to be able to tell people that I donated $100 in charity to Doris Duke. I must admit sending that letter really tickled me.

At about this point, Mrs. Cromwell, who had been in Hawaii, returned and must have gotten wind of the whole donnybrook because I received a check for the $100 difference from her New York office.

The last laugh was on Cromwell, who thought I'd never be allowed in the Duke house again. Actually, I treated her cats regularly in New York City for another twenty-four years. She'd call me in just to clip the cats' nails if nothing else was needed. When the Siamese were gone, I took care of one of the farm cats, who would be brought into town to see me. I outlasted James Cromwell in Doris Duke's life by several years, and I didn't miss him one minute of that time.

Chapter 14

IF I HAD MY WAY, every cat would have a home, but not the same home. While I can't give an exact figure for how many cats I approve of living in one residence, there is a cutoff point. Sometimes an accumulation of cats can become a burden which can create a difficult situation for some people. I don't say that *all* cat lovers should be limited in the number of cats they take in, but when a new pet is added, they should make certain they can care for it adequately without neglecting the ones already there.

I strongly advise people who are away from home all day to have two cats in their apartment instead of one. No one likes to be alone day after day, and that goes for cats, too.

The single cat will often show his displeasure at being abandoned daily. He may mess the owner's bed, tear things up, unravel the toilet paper, dig up potted plants, knock favorite knickknacks off shelves, and so on. You can quit your job and stay home or you can get a second cat.

Dolores Kreisman, a research psychologist, told me that every time she stayed out later than usual—or later than Smitty, her all-white domestic wanted her to—he would urinate on her bed. But when she brought Kissy Face, a dark-brown kitten, into the household and got Smitty to accept her, this behavior stopped.

Not that Smitty was ever truly wild about Kissy Face, but the presence of another cat gave him something to think about aside from when someone was coming home to pay attention to him.

A two-cat household has to be a little more carefully run. The cats should have their own bowls and be trained to stick to them. Phyllis Levy, the Books and Fiction Editor of *Ladies Home Journal,* not only trained her Barnaby and Tulip to eat from their own bowls, but also worked out a simple and effective system to know who was and who was not eating. One cat has his bowl on the floor, the other on the counter. If either cat goes off his or her feed, a possible sign of illness, Phyllis has only to keep an eye on the bowls to know.

A two-cat household also means twice as much combing, twice as much shedding, and twice as many litter box changes, but it is still better than one cat being alone most of the time.

The easiest way of having a two-cat household is to acquire both cats at the same time, and as kittens. There will probably be a few minor spats while the two cats work out the question of dominance, but since both cats have arrived at the same time, neither can have the feeling that his territory has been invaded by an outsider.

Introducing a second cat into an established one-cat household can be tricky, but it can be done. It just takes time and patience. I recommend separating the two cats by doors for several days, or even a few weeks if that seems necessary, until the cats get used to each other's presence. Switch them around occasionally, putting A into B's territory and B into A's so they can become accustomed to each other's smells. (This same method works just as well if you want to introduce a cat and a dog to each other.)

While the suggested method of introduction is a sound one, that doesn't mean it always works so simply. The very fine actress Barbara Baxley had a one-cat household until she saw someone abusing a black-and-white kitten. Without stopping to think whether or not she wanted a second cat, Barbara simply picked her up, named her Isabel on the spot and announced,

"If you don't like it, I shall report you to the ASPCA, Dr. Camuti and everyone else!" With that, she turned and took Isabel home.

By the time she reached home, Barbara realized she had acted strictly on impulse, without thinking. She had just returned from the national tour of *Dark at the Top of the Stairs* and hadn't gotten her own life in order without having to face the problem of trying to get two cats used to each other. Tula had been the sole cat in her life for some time and wasn't about to share the apartment or Barbara with some strange cat. Barbara knew that if they were left alone together Tula would kill Isabel.

She kept them in separate rooms and assumed that with time Tula would get used to the idea and the smell of Isabel. She was wrong. There was absolutely no decrease in Tula's hostility toward the stranger she smelled but never saw.

I finally suggested to Barbara that she have a screen door built into her apartment so the two cats would at least look at each other. She had one installed between the bedroom and the living room. The screen door took a beating for quite a while. Tula, having seniority, slept with Barbara as she always had, but Barbara, after first removing Isabel to safety, put Tula into the living room several times a day so that she could get accustomed to Isabel's having been there. During these times, Isabel enjoyed the bedroom and the adjacent balcony, Tula's territory.

It took several months, but finally the screen door was opened and peace was made. Tula immediately took charge as top cat and Isabel went along with it.

In case anyone is feeling sorry for Isabel as one of life's victims —first at the hands of the man Barbara Baxley rescued her from, and then by the dominance of Tula—don't. Isabel was not a cat with a docile nature. In fact, she was a tough cookie. That period of mistreatment in her youth had psychologically scarred her for life. I remember that after I had spayed Isabel and came to the apartment to remove the stitches that cat nearly killed both Barbara and me. Isabel hated to be touched, and it was nearly impossible to hold her to remove the stitches. She scratched and bit both of us until we had to release her. We had to turn the apartment upside down to find her to finish the job.

Much later, after Tula and Isabel had both died, a second pair of cats entered Barbara Baxley's life, but this pair was an entirely different story.

The first cat was Mr. Fay Wray, who was left to her by a friend when he died along with a small inheritance to pay for Mr. Fay's expenses.

Mr. Fay was the head—and only—cat in Barbara's life, or so she thought. Mr. Fay changed all that when he met a little cutie at Barbara's country place. Kiki simply walked in out of the woods, decided she liked Mr. Fay, the house, and Barbara, and that was that. No screen door was necessary this time, since the arrangement was of the cats' own choosing.

As the number of cats increases in a household, I am told that the pleasures increase, too. Maybe so. But there is also an increase in the number of food dishes that have to be put out and the number of litter pans that have to be changed. There's no single description for these people who have over a dozen cats —and I have had clients with as many as fifty cats. If they have anything in common, it is that their hearts are too big for their own good, because what they are doing can only be called self-sacrifice. They have so many mouths to feed and pans to clean that they have to give up a social life to get home the minute they leave their jobs. Whether they will admit it or not, these people are working for their cats all the time.

At this very moment, I have several clients who live with twenty-five to thirty cats in brownstone houses in Manhattan and in private homes in Brooklyn and the suburbs.

These people don't call me to see a different cat every week, because the sheer numbers they house make it impossible to notice which cat is off his feed, or is not eliminating properly, or isn't as playful as usual. Living that way, they can't be aware of the slight changes that reveal when a cat is going from well to sick. I often ask some of the ladies, "Could you be married to fifteen husbands?" It's the same thing. There is just so much time and so much concern one can give each day.

Finally, there is one other problem that is a part of all multiple-cat homes, and it is unsolvable. The smell. No matter how often an owner changes the litter and cleans the pans, too many cats do create a smell that eventually sinks into the rugs, the furniture and the drapes, probably even into the walls. But it is obviously worth it to those who live with and love their cats.

However, some may question whether so many cats being sheltered and fed together is better for them than having to live by their wits in the streets. Cats are creatures highly susceptible to disease, and if one cat takes ill, chances are that the disease will go through the whole house like wildfire.

One of my clients was a lady with a special fondness for Siamese cats. She had over two dozen of them, and each was named for a flower.

Though she didn't expect it, I did—the day came when she telephoned to tell me that all of her cats were sick. I went over to give them shots.

I set myself up in her kitchen, and she began bringing them in, one Siamese at a time. I gave shots to Pansy, Petunia, Daisy, Marigold, Violet, Rose, Lily, Daffodil, and for all I know, Stinkweed. Finally I called a halt as the woman came into the kitchen with another Siamese in her arms. "Whoa," I said, "just how many cats do you have?"

"Twenty-seven."

I looked at her. "Well, this is my thirty-second syringe. You've brought some of them in twice!"

They all looked alike, and it was impossible to recognize them, even though she thought she did. For all either of us could be certain, some of her Siamese could have gotten two and three shots, and others none.

So we worked out a system which I put into practice on my next visit. Each cat would get his or her shot and then a dab of lipstick on a different place each time I went to see them. Once it would be the ear, the next time the tail. That way I could be certain every cat was getting medical attention.

For this woman, and I think for many women, this multiplicity of cats represents an exaggerated form of the maternal instinct.

To me as a doctor, these women—and the men, too—always look exhausted. They come home from working all day and then are up half the night cleaning dishes and litter pans and putting out clean food dishes and clean litter. They are living on a feline treadmill. I often tell them, "Livestock is work twenty-four hours a day seven days a week and you can never say, 'I'll do it tomorrow' "—but these dedicated people don't listen.

And very often these people suffer for their love. Because of the smell that invariably accumulates—and there is no such thing as a deodorizing litter when you've got too many cats—there are many landlords who won't rent to them. Though these people might be able to afford good apartments in good neighborhoods, they are often forced to live on the periphery of the better neighborhoods unless they own their own homes.

I knew a Manhattan couple who lived for many years in a small, dark apartment, though they could have afforded more elegant quarters. But they could not find a landlord who would accept them with their twelve cats. Rather than get rid of any of their cats, they settled in and added a dog, a monkey and an aquarium filled with fish.

They lived with this menagerie in a one-room apartment, and the cats, naturally, were in charge. They picked the best sleeping places and continuously booted out the dog after he'd warmed up a spot one of them decided to use.

To save a little space, the couple rigged a pulley system from the ceiling with a cage for the monkey, who adjusted to living overhead.

Since the pulley system worked out so well, they added some Rube Goldberg contraptions for the cats: suspended platforms, swinging shelves and elevated snoozing compartments.

The cats loved it all. They could climb up high to check out the monkey, ambush each other from the suspended platforms, and play all sorts of cat games. To me, the place looked like a cross between a full-rigged schooner and backstage at the Metropolitan Opera.

Somehow everybody survived the clutter. Eventually the couple moved to a house in the suburbs along with their entire zoo. I don't know why I thought things would change when they got someplace that had more than one room. It didn't. All the contraptions had proved so successful in the one-room apartment that the couple took them with them, and with more room to work in added still more contraptions and gizmos. By the time I paid my first house call I thought I was walking through a giant Erector set.

Mr. and Mrs. Roland looked like a perfectly normal middle-aged couple living in a pleasant house with a yard that backed onto a woods. Unless you looked into their pantry, you would assume they didn't have any cats. But if you did look, you would wonder how many cats they owned because shelf after shelf was lined three deep in cat-food cans.

The Rolands told me that they didn't really think of themselves as "having" cats. "They're never in the house," Mrs. Roland explained.

What had happened was that a stray showed up one day at the back door, and they fed it. They fed it again the second day, and on the third day they saw the cat come out of the woods followed by a second cat. From that moment on, the word was out over the rural cat network, "Good grub at the Rolands." Before they knew it, the Rolands were buying their cat food by the case.

But none of the cats were ever invited inside the house. Neither Mr. nor Mrs. Roland ever named any of the cats or played with them, so they honestly didn't think of themselves as cat people. They were grateful to the cats for getting rid of so many of the moles that burrowed through their lawn, and the cats appreciated the pie pans filled with food that Mrs. Roland lined up in the backyard every day.

The problem arose when the Rolands decided to sell their house. They showed the real-estate brokers through the house and thought they seemed impressed. Unfortunately, the last broker came at cat suppertime. He happened to be looking out the rear window of the house as first one cat, then two more, came strolling out of the woods. He asked the Rolands if the cats were theirs.

"Not really," Mrs. Roland said. "They just eat here."

She got her pie pans and began filling them with cat food. By the time she had finished, more than a dozen cats were standing outside.

The real-estate man beat a hasty retreat, and word rapidly got around the neighborhood that there was "a bunch of wild cats" that "belonged" to the Rolands' place. It discouraged several potential buyers.

But one man showed up and expressed interest in the house. Unfortunately he made the mistake of telling the broker who brought him that the cats didn't bother him. If he decided on the house he would just put out poison or shoot the cats and that would be the end of that. Mrs. Roland overheard him and refused to sell him the house.

Their sense of responsibility to the cats was so great that the Rolands decided to take the house off the market. They realized that they had grown quite fond of the cats and that much of their life pivoted around feeding time and seeing the cats appear. And they knew that the cats had come to depend on them. If they were just a few minutes late in putting out the food pans there would be a racket from the gathering throng. Once they had eaten, the cats stayed around only long enough to wash up. Then they drifted silently back into the woods until the next afternoon.

At one point Mr. and Mrs. Roland counted twenty cats of varied colors and sizes waiting in the garden for the pans to come out. Then suddenly the number started thinning down.

Since there was no change in the area in which they lived, the Rolands were at a loss to explain what was happening. Yet, within a few weeks, there were less than eight cats showing up, then six, and then one night there were no more cats.

Mrs. Roland couldn't believe the cats were getting better dinners from someone else. She continued to put out a few pie pans and call to the cats. But no one came. After a few days she gave up.

To the Rolands the disappearance of the cats seemed like a mystery. But I think there must have been an epidemic, such as infectious enteritis, that spread through the colony. As each animal sickened it crept off deep into the woods to die. But without searching the woods—and neither of the Rolands had the heart for that—there was no way of knowing for sure.

With the cats gone, the Rolands put the house back on the market. They said it was too lonely.

They had no trouble selling.

Chapter 15

I IMAGINE that there are doctors who at some point in their careers tire of their specialty, but I doubt that I ever will. There are too many surprises when your patients are cats. Just when I think I've seen everything a cat can do, along comes one who upsets the applecart.

If I've ever had a hard-and-fast rule about cats in general it is that they all run and hide when Camuti rings the doorbell. And if there's a second rule it's that they disappear after I've finished with them and they stay out of sight until I'm long gone. And yet, I can think of an exception to each of those rules.

Chiula was a Siamese who lived with May Lamberton Becker, a delightful lady who wrote childrens' books as well as a column for the old *Tribune*. Mrs. Becker lived in a cooperative apartment on Morningside Drive, and whenever I went up there to see Chiula or one of the lady Siamese Mrs. Becker provided for him as a mate, there was Chiula at the door to greet me. He would rub against my leg and walk me into the apartment, talking a steady stream all the way. And if I had come to see one of Chiula's wives or kittens Chiula hung around until I was through. The minute I released my patient, who promptly shot out of the kitchen, Chiula went into his act, crying and rubbing and throwing himself on his back until I got the message that he wanted to be examined, too. Sometimes I'd pretend not to see him and begin to pack my bag. That was the cue for Chiula to howl louder and roll around on the floor, taking nips at my pants legs until I noticed him. Then I'd make a great fuss of looking in his ears and patting his chest and stomach while he purred in contentment.

When the so-called examination was over, Chiula would puff out his chest and strut around the apartment with a great show of pride. It really made my day to have a cat look forward to seeing me.

If Chiula was an exceptional patient, he was also a very passionate husband and an affectionate father. He kept Mrs. Becker hopping to supply him with mates. Sure as clockwork, Chiula sired three litters a year by each of his wives, all of whom were so worn out at the end of three years that Mrs. Becker would have to go out and find a new female for Chiula.

If I hadn't seen Chiula with his kittens I wouldn't have believed it. According to everything I know, male cats are not particularly interested in their young. Usually they have no family instincts beyond the urge to mate. Having kittens is entirely the female's job.

But Chiula took a great interest in his sons and daughters. Often when I'd stop off to check on a new litter, I'd see Chiula boot the mother out of her bed if he felt she was nursing too long. Then he'd take her place and curl up with the kittens. When he had enough of parental responsibility he would look over to the mother and let her know it was time to come back.

There was only one time that Chiula was less than a perfect cat. It was when Mrs. Becker had to go to see her daughter in England just at the time that Chiula's current wife, Lucia, was expecting a litter. I told Mrs. Becker I would care for Chiula and see Lucia through her delivery at my hospital. And I said I would put Lucia in a separate cage when her labor began since it is not unusual for the male to kill the kittens.

"I don't think that's a good idea," Mrs. Becker said. "Chiula's so accustomed to being with his mate that it might upset him. I don't want to sound hardhearted, but I'd rather lose the kittens than upset Chiula."

I didn't believe that any tom would be upset by the temporary absence of his female, so when her moment came I removed Lucia from the cage she shared with Chiula and put her in a separate one nearby.

Chiula didn't like it one bit. He stopped eating and began yowling. He paced and cried, and reached out to Lucia through the bars.

Lucia, meanwhile, delivered five healthy kittens and was totally engrossed in caring for them.

The birth of the kittens made things even worse for Chiula. He became more anxious, still refused to eat and cried endlessly.

After a few days of his unrelenting misery, Lucia took up the cry. Neither of them were doing themselves, each other, the kittens—or me—any good. I decided Mrs. Becker was right. They needed to be together. The continuous crying convinced me that the new kittens would probably survive a return of Chiula to Lucia's cage.

The reunion was wildly affectionate with lots of sniffing, licking and purring. And they even showed some interest in the food bowls again.

But in the morning, all five kittens were gone. There was no way to know if Chiula or Lucia or both of them were responsible. But both cats were content and asleep, curled up together.

To this day I wonder if it was the cages, the foreign environment of my hospital or something that Chiula—and maybe Lucia—knew about that one litter. Certainly it had never happened before with the litters Chiula had sired, and it never happened again with all the litters Chiula fathered by Lucia and his other wives. And all the litters that followed saw Chiula offering the same parental concern he always exhibited—in Mrs. Becker's apartment.

It seems appropriate to report the circumstance of Chiula's death. He was in the middle of mating with his sixth wife when he just toppled over.

As for the cat that doesn't disappear when I've finished with him, that distinction goes to Barnaby, one of Phyllis Levy's two tabby Persians. I see a great deal of Barnaby and Tulip since they both suffer with the same chronic upper-respiratory infection that requires my giving them thrice-weekly shots to keep their condition controlled. And if either catches a cold, I see them daily. If Phyllis were any less devoted to her cats she'd have returned them to the cat store after my first examination. But in each case, it was love at first sight, and so we've gone on like this year after year.

The treatment routine is always the same, and the behavior of the two tabbies is, too. Tulip hides in the closet when she hears me at the apartment door. Phyllis lets me in, then gets Tulip out of the closet. I give her her shot in the kitchen, after which Tulip runs back into the closet.

Barnaby takes his shot like a man, and only runs away for a minute. What follows after that is what makes Barnaby unique. He throws me out of the apartment.

When I finish with her cats, I take a break in my routine to have a cup of tea with Phyllis. Three times a week we sit down at her Parsons table, in exactly the same place facing each other. We barely get in two sips of tea when Barnaby comes into the room.

He sits down between us facing the front door, his back to us and his tail twitching impatiently. At this point, both Phyllis and I start gulping our tea because we know what's coming. And if we have anything important to say, we know it's now or never.

After a few minutes of tail twitching, a hint from Barnaby that I refuse to take, he gets up and comes to stand in front of me, making low but audible cat noises. At this point, Phyllis and I can still hear each other so we go on with our conversation. But the cat noises turn into yowls that grow louder and louder as Barnaby starts pacing back and forth between us with mounting agitation. Finally, conversation is impossible and I have to leave. Barnaby's performance takes place three times a week every week.

I don't call him Barnaby. Bastardo is my name for him, and so far, he has never told me what he calls me. But I'll bet it's a beauty.

Chapter 16

IT'S A RARE WEEK that goes by that I don't get a letter about some cat who performs a marvelous trick. And about once a month I'll visit a client who will insist on showing me what his cat can do. The trouble is the cat rarely does whatever it is he "always" does. All I ever get out of the performance which doesn't take place is a waste of my time.

Cats, as a general rule, are not performers the way dogs are. It's not that they can't learn—cats are more than bright enough —it's that they can't be bothered to learn. To sit up and beg the way a dog will or to roll over and play dead is beneath a cat's dignity—silly human stuff to be ignored unless it somehow suits the cat's purpose.

I've run into an occasional trained cat and I've seen them in television commercials, but how they are lured to eat their crunchies on cue is something I don't want to know about.

One of the things that made me decide against accepting performing cats as patients is the impression that their owners were more concerned with money than with their cats' welfare. I remember being called in to treat a white cat that was appearing in a Broadway show. Someone at the theater decided that the cat didn't look white enough on stage because it was picking up backstage dirt. Every day, and I assume twice on matinee days, that poor cat was given a bath to keep it spotless. As any cat lover knows, cats do the best cleaning jobs by themselves. No one has to bathe a cat. It was no wonder to me that that white longhair got sick. Whoever bathed him didn't dry him well enough, and the stage was probably drafty. When I told this to the cat's owner, I could see his eyes glaze over. He wasn't interested. So I got hold of the stage manager of the show and laced into him. That was when I swore off treating professional cats.

While cats are not always successful as performers, they are marvelous trainers of people. In almost no time at all, a cat can teach its owner that a certain flip of the tail means "follow me" as it leads the way to an empty food bowl or to the closed garden door. Likewise, people learn very quickly that a meow in the face, a lick on the ankles or a bottle knocked off a bureau means "Get up, you lazy good-for-nothing and feed me." The owner, in turn, will then rave to his friends about the marvelous trick his cat performs, but the cat knows who has taught whom.

I remember a letter from a woman in Australia who lived on a farm where her cat learned to pull a bell cord and ring the porch bell when it wanted to come indoors. If the woman didn't come running fast enough, the cat would leap onto one of the porch rocking chairs and rock it against the side of the house. That thumping was a sound the lady couldn't miss hearing.

Marilyn and Hank Frankel's cat, Balaban, really hasn't any tricks in his repertoire—but he did have a mad crush on Gregory Peck. Hank is a late-show addict, and whenever he watched a film with Gregory Peck in it, Balaban came running to curl up on the table ledge on which the set rested while Gregory Peck was in the scene. For those scenes, Hank could only listen to the movie because Balaban blocked out a large part of the screen. If Mr. Peck was not in the next scene, Balaban immediately lost interest and went back to whatever he was doing, only to reappear the next time he heard the Peck voice. Hank isn't certain whether it was maturity or Balaban's neutering that changed everything, but today he is no longer interested in Gregory Peck.

Frederico was a cat with even more decided television preferences than Balaban. According to a Miss Winters who wrote to me about him, Frederico had an aversion to Art Linkletter. Whenever he heard Mr. Linkletter's voice, Frederico came running into the room and pushed the button that shut off the set.

Frederico had one trick, self-taught, that would stop traffic in the streets whenever he did it. Frederico would search the house for cigarette butts. When he found one, he'd lounge on his side in the window, the butt hanging from his mouth.

I would imagine that anyone who ever saw Lily-boy, the love of Judy Lynn Prince's childhood, would have thought him a professional cat or at least a trained one. But as far as I am concerned Lily-boy was just very tolerant.

Lily-boy was the kitten of Foundit. Foundit, as you can tell from her name, was lost. And was found pregnant. Lily-boy was the only kitten from her litter that the Princes kept. Lily was the name Judy Lynn always wanted for a cat, so when her all-black kitten turned out to be a male, she just tacked "-boy" onto the end.

From his tiniest kitten days, Lily-boy was Judy Lynn's and she was his, and they both knew it. Daily she would dress him up in doll clothes, sit him in a doll carriage and parade him around the yard. Surprisingly enough, Lily-boy never protested. In fact, hat on head and wearing a large-size doll's dress, he sat up proud in his carriage.

Lily-boy even accepted invitations—through Judy Lynn—to child-size tea parties. Judy Lynn would put him in a chair at the tea table and he stayed there. About the only rule of etiquette he broke was when he leaned forward to lick his milk out of his saucer.

The question is did Lily-boy put up with all of this because Judy Lynn had trained him—and could a child succeed where adult trainers have failed?—or is it simply that Lily-boy enjoyed it all and knew that this nonsense paid off in extra treats that cats who refused to attend tea parties didn't get?

Few cats fetch, but Tula, Barbara Baxley's cat, did. It wasn't a trick, but a game that Tula chose to play. But there was only one person Tula would play fetch with. That was Donald Cook, the well-known actor, whom she considered her best friend, next to Barbara. It was frustrating to Barbara that no matter how often she would crumple the cigarette Cellophane and toss it just the way that Donald Cook did, Tula didn't respond. She merely looked where the Cellophane landed and went on with whatever she was or wasn't doing. But let Donald Cook appear and crumple the Cellophane, and the game was on.

I will concede to one trained cat in all my experience. That was Beebe, a female Siamese, who lived with Earle Larimore, a fine Broadway actor during the '20s and '30s, and his actress wife, Selena Royle. Since they both worked with great frequency, but usually in different plays, I would see one or the other of them whenever I made a house call for Beebe.

If Mr. Larimore was home I groaned, because I knew I was in for a performance by one of the few "trick cats" in the history of show business. And frankly I didn't relish it, because I had seen the performance a dozen times before. But that never stopped Earle Larimore.

If it didn't happen at the beginning of a visit to their apartment in the East 50's, it happened at the end. Mr. Larimore would say, "Dr. Camuti, do you want to see the bumps game?"

It got to the point where I'd say outright, "Mr. Larimore, I've seen it a hundred times!"

That didn't bother him at all. "Okay, we'll show you again. Positions everyone!"

Beebe would go to one corner of the room and Earle Larimore would go to the opposite corner. "Let's play bumps," he'd shout to the cat. That was her cue to stalk toward him, as slowly as if she were out in the woods stalking wild game. Earle Larimore would get down on his hands and knees and approach Beebe in the same manner while I'd sit glancing at my watch and tapping my foot as man and cat slowly approached each other. I'd have to remind myself that the fanny I was looking at in the expensive trousers belonged to a man who had performed with the Lunts and appeared in Theatre Guild premiere productions of Eugene O'Neill plays.

Finally, when Beebe and Earle Larimore met each other in the middle of the living room, they would both look up and bump heads.

I wouldn't even make a move to get up. I knew the performance wasn't over. Earle Larimore would stand up, brush his trousers at the knees, and then call to the Siamese, "Beebe, go Hollywood!" Beebe would immediately drop to the floor, roll over on her back and thrash her legs in the air in some bizarre, imagined cat orgy. No matter how many times I saw that one, I always had to laugh at the sight of that dignified Siamese flailing about on her back.

Beebe had one more trick, and it is one I've never seen anyone else do with a cat. Earle Larimore would make a circle with his two arms and Beebe would lower her head, get a running start and leap through the "hoop."

If Earle Larimore hadn't been such a successful actor, I think he and Beebe could have made it as an act in the heyday of vaudeville or maybe even the circus. Of course, I'd have had to see him train another cat to do Beebe's tricks to know that Earle Larimore had a magic touch as a cat trainer. After all, it could have been that the right cat came along, one with a streak of ham in him.

To look at Joe, who is also known as Boots, you might think he was just another gray-and-white striped domestic shorthair. He's the cat I told you about whom Tom and Alice Fleming, the writers, put in a closet of their summer house with a mouse, only to have both come out in the same shape in which they entered.

But in his younger days Joe was one of the great feline athletes of his time, champion player of both football and baseball in the Flemings' New York apartment.

Joe's passion for football dates back to when the Flemings' three sons were in grammar school. Their football field was the long hallway that ran the length of the apartment from the living room down to their bedroom. What began as a three-man game became a one-against-three game when Joe decided to join in.

The boys would huddle with the ball in the living room. At the sound of the boys shouting signals from the huddle Joe would take his position in the hallway, lurking in one of the doorways. The shout of "Hike" was Joe's cue to get into defensive position with his front end low and his hindquarters trembling. When the home team came crashing down the hallway, Joe went into action. With the prowess of a Rosie Greer, Joe tackled the ball carrier, who'd fall to the floor—he'd have to because Joe wouldn't let go of his leg—yelling, "Ya got me, Joe, ya got me!" That was Joe's signal to release the ball carrier.

The boys would regroup for a new rush to the bedroom goal, and Joe would get back into a doorway again. And again he would fly out to tackle the ball carrier. To the best of anyone's memory no one ever scored against Joe. He could play the game for an hour and not tire of it. The boys usually gave out long before Joe was ready to quit.

He was also an admirable baseball player—a switch hitter. The Flemings always knew when Joe felt like a couple of innings because he would step into his batter's box which was the bottom shelf of the bookcase. Then one of the Flemings would toss a crumpled piece of paper to him and Joe would hit at it.

The Fleming boys worked out a score system for Joe. A hit to the coffee table was a single, as far as the chair was a double, and to the sofa was a home run.

But the years have passed and the boys have become men and moved away from home. Joe's gotten older too, but there's no doubt that he remembers and misses the old days. Alice Fleming can testify to it. Every now and then, when she returns from marketing at D'Agostino's and is heading down the hall toward the kitchen with a full bag of groceries, Joe comes flying out of a doorway and tackles her.

Chapter 17

TREATING CATS and caring for them have certainly been my lifework, but let's not ignore the people they live with. They fascinate me. When I get a call to see a cat that might or might not have ringworm, I know I am going to see a cat that does or does not have ringworm. It's as simple as that. But I don't know what kind of household I'm going into or what kind of people I am going to be dealing with. That's where the fun and excitement comes into my work.

And that's why I say that some people are more normal than others. The way I work has taken me to every corner of New York City—rich and poor—and into an awful lot of the surrounding territory, and that means I have met a great many people. And while most of them, I am sure, are quite sensible in other areas of their lives, something seems to happen to them when it comes to their relationships with their cats.

Don't get me wrong. I'm not trying to explain some of the people I've come in contact with in terms of a cat setting them off. Some of them would have been just as wacky if they'd been living with a pet turtle. The only difference is that I wouldn't have run into them.

Like the ballet dancer who called me to come see her cat, and turned out to be a cleanliness nut. She met me at the door of her apartment and told me to take off my shoes. Well, I could look past her and see through the open door at what was going on inside. She had her chairs, sofa and even her rugs covered in plastic. I decided right then and there that the lady was a bit off. I like things to be clean, too, but I know you don't create a sterile atmosphere just by having people remove their shoes. I told the woman I was going to keep my shoes on and she could keep her cat. With that I turned and left.

There was a rich woman in Rye, New York, who was also a cleanliness nut—well, maybe I'm being unfair to her. Maybe I turned her into one when I first saw her sick cat and told her to keep everything as clean as possible around the cat. All I know is that when I later came on house calls, she'd have the house-man answer the door wearing white cotton gloves. The lady herself would come to greet me carrying a can of spray disinfec-tant, which she used on the doorknob. She'd follow me from room to room in the house spraying doorknobs and wiping them off.

When her cat finally died, she took the furniture and the rug from the cat's room and had it stacked in the center of her backyard where she burned all of it. I tried to tell the woman that her cat's illness could only have been contagious to other cats—and she had none—not to people. She just nodded her head and put a match to everything.

Generally, I find doctors and nurses make the worst clients, but don't ask me why. You'd think they'd be accustomed to medical procedures and the sight of blood, but it just isn't so when it comes to their own cat. Dr. John Prutting, who has been my personal physician since 1947, would always find an excuse not to be home when I was coming to treat his cat.

Years ago, when I had my office at 65 Park Avenue, George Mosby came in and said, "The man who's your next appoint-ment insists on staying to watch while you spay his cat."

"Throw him out," I said. "He's not telling me what to do. Absolutely not."

In those days I didn't consider having nonmedical people hovering over my patients, asking questions and in general interfering with my work. Of course, when I switched my practice to house calls I tried to get my clients to help me, or I'd have Alex come in and work with me.

George went out to tell the client that I wouldn't permit him in the office while I was spaying his cat. But George was back a minute or two later, shaking his head. "The man insists, Doctor."

"Okay, I'll handle it." I went out into the waiting room. The man stood up as I entered. He was over six feet tall and built like a heavyweight.

"Just what sort of work do you do?" I asked him.

"I'm a slaughterer in a slaughterhouse."

That changed everything for me. "Then it's okay. You're certainly used to the sight of blood. I'll let you watch, but don't say anything."

He agreed and I took him into the hospital room and sat him on a bench in a corner while I scrubbed up.

When I anesthetized the cat, I turned to the man. "Now, I want you to understand that there'll be a certain sound when I slice the skin, and there may be a spurt of blood when we go a little further. . . ."

The man just nodded. "It's okay. I told you I slaughter cattle all day."

So I began, but I kept taking peeps at the man in the corner. As I cut through the second layer of tissue I could see that he was turning chalk white. But I had warned him.

I didn't even look up when I heard the groan followed by a thump as he hit the floor.

George was going to go to the man, who was out cold, but I felt our duty was to the patient. "The hell with him. Let him stay there," I said to George.

After the cat was sewn up and resting, George and I lifted the man to his feet. He looked sheepish as he tried to apologize. "Forget it," I said. "Save it for the gang at the slaughterhouse."

Years ago, there were certain medications we used that, truth to tell, worked better in the hospital than in the home. One of them was Neo-Prontosil, a sulfur drug that predated antibiotics as a treatment for infection. It worked well, but the trouble with the stuff was that it turned all the visible membranes of the cat red, and when the body voided it hours later the urine was bright red too. I used the stuff once to teach a lesson to a client.

Her name was Nila Mack. She was the creator of the famous children's radio show, "Let's Pretend." While I can't remember why I was treating her cat with a series of shots, I do remember that I had to see him several days in a row.

I arrived one afternoon and there was Nila Mack, and she looked tense and angry. "Is everything all right?" I asked.

"It's about yesterday's injection," she said.

"Did the cat react to it?"

"That's just it," she said. "I don't think you gave him one."

"Well, you saw me with the syringe." I still thought she might be kidding, so I added, "Fastest shot in the East they call me."

But she didn't smile. "I know all that, but he didn't flinch or anything. I don't know what to think."

Well, I couldn't have a prominent person like Nila Mack thinking I was a fraud. So that day, when I gave her cat his usual shot, I added a dose of Neo-Prontosil.

In a few hours my telephone rang. It was Nila Mack, and she was hysterical. "My cat's bleeding to death!"

I knew exactly what was wrong with her cat, but I said I'd be right over. All I needed was one quick look at the cat and its litter box to know that the Neo-Prontosil had done its work. I calmed Nila Mack down and explained to her what I had done and why I had done it. "I couldn't have you thinking that Camuti was a gyp artist," I said.

She, of course, apologized.

Another medicine that caused a hubbub was gentian violet. The client was Penny Willis, who lived at the Beaux Arts Hotel near the United Nations. Penny was a nice, sweet lady who was always falling in love with a new man, and when Penny was in love, everything else went right out of her head.

One day Penny called me to say that she thought Finley, her Siamese, had ringworm. I said I'd stop by.

As I went to work on Finley with the ultraviolet lamp and the Woods filter, a contraption that makes the hair show green where ringworm is, I glanced over at Penny and saw that vague, faraway stare that told me she was in love again.

Finley had ringworm all right. I showed Penny where the spots were and gave her some gentian violet with instructions on how to use the stuff. I gave Finley the first application myself and told Penny that all she had to do was reapply the gentian violet periodically to those few places and Finley would soon be cured. Penny nodded absent-mindedly.

To make sure she was paying attention, I said, "Now, remember. You put the gentian violet only on those spots I showed you. Gentian violet can be toxic, and cats usually try to lick the stuff off."

A few days later, when I went back to the hotel to check on my patient, the desk clerk said, "Tell me, Doc, have you ever seen a purple cat?"

I told him there was no such thing.

"That's what I thought," the clerk said, "but I wanted you to confirm it. You know, we have several banquet rooms that we rent out for business meetings and so on. Well, a few days ago, the bell captain got a call from one of those rooms that there was a purple cat in the hall. We didn't pay much attention to it. We figured the men in that room had too many cocktails with their lunch. But about five minutes later, we got a call from a different room requesting that a bellman come up and remove a purple cat."

The clerk looked at me, waiting for me to say something. I kept quiet, but I had a pretty darn good idea what was going on.

"Anyway," the clerk said, "we sent a man up, but of course there was no cat in the room. But what we've been wondering is how two separate groups could have the same hallucination. What do you think?"

"Beats me," I said and headed for Penny Willis's apartment.

The minute I saw Finley, indeed a purple cat, I wanted to wring Penny's neck, but I felt sorry for her. I knew how much she loved Finley so she wouldn't have risked his life unless her latest love affair was going very badly. And judging from her red eyes, it was.

As for Finley, why he wasn't dead I'll never figure out. His entire body was purple, and his tongue was denuded of tissue from licking at himself. While it took only about a month to cure Finley's ringworm, it took me three months to get his tongue back into shape.

The only odd thing about Florence Piper was her cat, Linn, a seal-point Siamese. Miss Piper was a gentle and loving lady, an absolute pleasure to have for a client. Linn was something else again, a cat who hated every living thing on the face of this earth including me and sometimes Miss Piper. Now why would anyone want to live with a cat like that?

The answer had to be love. Miss Piper had acquired Linn as a kitten from a home in which he had obviously been badly mistreated. When she took Linn to her house in Flushing, Miss Piper gave the kitten lots of love, but it wasn't enough to erase the scars buried deep within Linn.

By the time Linn grew up and proved to be vicious, Miss Piper loved him too much to consider getting rid of him. She found herself living with a cat who wouldn't allow anyone except his owner to pet him, and even her only on rare occasions.

She couldn't let Linn have the run of her yard and expect him to come back when she called. In order for the cat to get any fresh air, Miss Piper had to put on a collar, a halter and two leashes to restrain him. Linn enjoyed his walks with her, but she could only take him out late at night because all hell would break loose when Linn encountered anyone—cat, dog or person.

Whenever Miss Piper wanted to entertain she'd have to put

Linn in the basement. Though it gave him a huge area in which to play he hated it. He'd spend most of his time at the top of the cellar stairs growling and spitting behind the door until the guest had left. There were no two ways about it, Linn altered and dominated Florence Piper's life.

One time Miss Piper's brother-in-law made the mistake of dropping by without calling first. Linn was asleep upstairs, and Miss Piper forgot about him while she bustled about making tea. While she was in the kitchen, Linn awakened and crept downstairs into the living room. He took one look at Miss Piper's brother-in-law and leaped for the man's throat. It took all of his efforts and Miss Piper's to get the cat away. The man's shirt was shredded, and his face, neck and chest were badly scratched.

Everyone in Miss Piper's world knew about Linn. The window cleaner was so afraid of Linn—actually, he was afraid of all cats —that he would telephone several times before he arrived at her house.

When he did show up, he would refuse to enter the house until Miss Piper assured him that Linn was locked up in the basement. One time, however, the basement door was insecurely shut. The window cleaner was at work on the inside of one of the windows and Miss Piper was elsewhere in the house when Linn got the basement door open. As the window cleaner later explained it, "It was spooky. I don't know how but I just felt the cat sneaking up on me."

He turned and saw Linn stalking him, body low to the ground, ears flat back, tail moving slowly from side to side. As the man watched in horror, Linn got into lunge position, his hindquarters wiggling for the pounce. There was only one possible escape for the window washer, and he took it. He dived head first through the closed window he'd been washing. The bursting wood and shattering glass brought Miss Piper on the run. Luckily, the man had been working on the ground floor.

He was bleeding so badly that he had to be rushed to the hospital. His cut-up throat, which required stitches, took over a week to heal. Miss Piper visited him several times, always telling him how sorry she was.

"Don't feel so bad," the man told her. "It would have been worse if the cat had gotten me."

Treating Linn was never an easy job. In fact, I only saw him awake once because Miss Piper and I had worked out a system. I would call her an hour before I expected to arrive at her house, and she would give Linn enough Nembutal to anesthetize him. Luckily he would let her give him the capsule without too much difficulty so that he was asleep by the time I arrived.

Once, however, he fooled both Miss Piper and me. As usual, when I arrived I asked, "Is he asleep?" and she said he was. But he wasn't. On that occasion, he had somehow slipped the pill into a corner of his mouth instead of swallowing it. Then he lay down for a catnap.

Not knowing it wasn't an anesthetized sleep, I went into the downstairs bedroom where she had placed Linn after giving him his pill. I started toward the cat to pick him up when he opened his eyes and glared at me. I knew exactly what he had in mind and I flew backward through the open doorway as he leaped. I slammed the door shut while Linn was in midair and heard him crash into it head on.

I didn't stop after closing the door, not with Linn in a rage on the other side. My adrenalin was racing, my heart was pounding and I started running. In the front hall I slipped on a scatter rug and fell, hitting my head against a table leg, which knocked me out cold.

Linn was not treated that night.

In time Linn developed a recurring bladder infection that necessitated my seeing him every other night for weeks at a time to express his urine by massaging his abdomen. That went on for five years, and I can't remember one visit to Linn when I had any feeling of the animal's gratitude to me for relieving its pressure and internal pain.

During all those years, it was always a question to me which one of us would go first. Luckily, it was the cat.

While I don't like to speak ill of the dead, there isn't much good I can remember about Linn except Miss Piper's love for him. Well, there was one thing, I guess.

Linn used to enjoy sitting in the front-porch window of Miss Piper's house watching people, especially children on their way to school. Linn would hiss, growl and spit at all of them so they could hear him through the screen. Eventually people stopped walking on Miss Piper's side of the street. What was good about this was that there came a time when there was a wave of burglaries in Miss Piper's neighborhood. Houses all around her were ransacked. But either the sight of Linn in the window or his reputation protected Miss Piper's house. It was never touched.

The Hartmans struck me as a charming and likable couple the first time I went to see their two cats, Mutt and Jeff. But as time went by, I saw Mrs. Hartman turn into a depressed and deeply disturbed woman. One night when I came to see the cats and her husband wasn't home she told me that she was certain her husband was seeing another woman. I didn't want to get involved with what was not my business but I had to say something, so I asked her what made her think so. All she could say was, "I just know. I feel it inside."

I could hardly put much belief in that statement as evidence of any sort, so I forgot about it, deciding that her fears were symptoms of some other problem.

In any case, I underestimated the depth of Mrs. Hartman's depression because one day I read in the newspaper that she had killed herself. It was horrible. She had put her head in the oven and turned on the gas. As the gas filled the apartment, the cats ran for the bedroom and with their natural instinct for survival crawled under a bureau where there was a pocket of clean air.

When Lily, the Hartman maid, arrived for work and rang the front doorbell, it created an electric spark that caused an explosion so great that it knocked down a kitchen wall.

While Mutt and Jeff survived the explosion, they got respiratory ailments as a result of the water the fire department poured into the apartment. Mr. Hartman called me to come over.

I went back again a few weeks later to check on my patients. I found Mr. Hartman looking drawn and tense, which seemed natural to me under the circumstances. At one point, he absent-mindedly picked up the cigar I had put down in an ashtray and started to smoke it.

There were several bouquets of flowers in the room. I assumed they were sent by friends after the funeral. I tried to say something consoling, but I wasn't much help. Tears came to his eyes and he began to moan, "My poor wife, my poor wife." He said it over and over again.

I waited for him to pull himself together. In the silence, I heard someone moving around in another room. I assumed it was Lily, and I was glad she hadn't quit him after the explosion. He looked like a man who shouldn't be left alone.

When he had collected himself, he said, "Forgive me, Doctor, there's someone I want you to meet."

He turned his head toward the room where I thought Lily was and called out, "Oh, dear, can you come in a moment?"

I knew he wasn't calling Lily, and I felt a chill crawl up my back. Mr. Hartman had cracked. He imagined his wife was still alive.

To my astonishment, a lovely young woman came into the room. Mr. Hartman stood up. "Dr. Camuti, I'd like you to meet my wife."

I have never been so astounded in my life. The first Mrs. Hartman had been right all along!

A top businesswoman who used to be a client of mine adored her two cats to the point where her private life completely revolved around them. At least, I think it did, since her apartment was decorated more to suit the cats than herself. While I admired what she had done with the place I couldn't quite picture her bringing home boyfriends or business associates to the apartment.

What she had done was to give her indoor cats all the fun of outdoors without any of the risks. Because all cats love to climb and sit on high places, she had two ladders—one for each cat—as a permanent part of her living room. They were standard stepladders that were painted to match the room and decorated with decals. The ledges where painters rest their paint cans made perfect sleeping places, and both of her cats knew it. These were their favorite places for a snooze.

She had two tables set up on either side of her fireplace with a board running across the fireplace from table to table making a bridge. The cats liked racing back and forth on it.

Then she bought them a dwarf apple tree, thinking they'd like to scratch on it. They didn't scratch, but instead began eating the leaves, so she gave me the tree. I took it out to my daughter in New Jersey where it still grows in her yard.

While the woman was very good about keeping her adored cats on the baby-beef diet I recommended, she did have one special treat for them. Seeing how much fun her cats had with a housefly, she hired her building superintendent's young son to catch five flies each day. He was to bring them to her apartment in a glass jar each morning before she went to work. She paid the boy one dollar per fly, and she released them in the apartment as she left for work, knowing the cats would play the flies to death and then eat them. She also figured she was giving her cats a lot of exercise at the same time.

One day, the superintendent came up with his son. "Don't you think the cats would have more fun with ten flies a day?"

My client assured him that five flies—and five dollars—a day was quite sufficient.

I lost track of the woman when she moved to California.

Mrs. Thorndyke was another lady who was devoted to her cats, two short-haired domestics. Mrs. Thorndyke lived in a large cooperative apartment on Central Park West. I was told by the friend who recommended me to her that Mrs. Thorndyke was considered an excellent hostess.

With her reputation, I wasn't surprised to arrive for a house call and see her dining table handsomely set for what looked like a child's party.

As she led me to the kitchen where the cat I was to treat was waiting she saw me glance at the table. "It's a birthday party," she said.

"For your granddaughter?" I asked.

She shook her head. "For the cats. I can never remember their birth dates so I make one party every year for the two of them."

With two cats and four places at the table, it wasn't too difficult for me to figure out the guest list. When I finished treating her cat, Mrs. Thorndyke led me back to the dining room. "Now, you sit there where your place card is. After all, you're their doctor. If anyone should be invited . . ."

I decided, Why not? I was ready for a break anyway.

I sat where I was told and while Mrs. Thorndyke went in search of the guests of honor, read the other place cards. The one I'd just given a shot to wasn't about to be social with me, and the other cat, dreading what might be in store for him with me still on the premises, went into hiding. Whenever Mrs. Thorndyke did catch one of the cats and sit him at the table he would jump off the chair the minute she let him go.

In time there were just Mrs. Thorndyke and me eating melted ice cream and watching candle wax drip onto the birthday cake. She apologized profusely. I told her it didn't matter, and that I'd be delighted to come back for next year's party.

I didn't tell Mrs. Thorndyke that I wasn't the least surprised at the way the birthday party turned out. I've been to dozens of cat parties and it's been a rare one at which a cat has chosen to stay. I've also attended cat funerals, cat wakes and cat weddings. And once I attended a cat's bar mitzvah.

Dr. and Dr. Katz, as I called them—since they were both medical people—asked me how to figure the age of their cat, Harry. I told them that the way I saw it, since the average well-cared-for person lives approximately seventy-five years, one calendar year would equal five cat years.

Two years after I neutered Harry—he was about six months old then—I got a call from the female Dr. Katz. She said that she and her husband had decided it was time for Harry's bar mitzvah. Would I attend? Since I hadn't known any cats who celebrated this passage into manhood, or cathood in Harry's case, I said I'd be delighted.

As bar mitzvahs go it wasn't much. We all sat around the table wearing yarmulkas, but the bar mitzvah boy never joined us. After a ceremonial glass of wine with the Katzes I left.

It's part of every doctor's job, mine included, to answer questions. I certainly don't mind taking the time to explain a cat's illness to a client, or to spell out proper care. But sometimes the questions get out of hand.

Today John Lahr is a pretty well-known writer and theater critic, but back when I knew him he was just a young shaver. He showed up with his dog, Barry, who had a unilateral nasal discharge, at my office on Park Avenue. I treated the dog for some time.

Sometimes John came with his mother; at other times his sister accompanied him. At the end of each visit John would always ask if I would mind calling his father that evening to explain everything to him. I said I'd be happy to. It pleased me that the whole family was concerned with the dog's health.

My telephone conversations with the father were usually lengthy ones as he always had many questions, and from the perceptiveness of his questions I could tell that he was a medical man.

After some time with this routine I ended a long conversation with Dr. Lahr by asking him what his medical specialty was.

He sounded astonished. "Specialty, what specialty? I'm an actor."

I had been talking to the famous actor-comedian Bert Lahr. The reason he knew so much about medicine was that he was a hypochondriac.

Sometimes you begin to wonder about clients you always thought of as solid citizens when they recommend you to friends of theirs who turn out to be nutty as fruitcakes.

I remember going to a very fine address on the recommendation of a very proper longtime client of mine. At the new client's place, the door was opened for me by a Japanese house-boy. The foyer looked impressive. The houseboy took me through the foyer and into the living room, where the new client was seated at the piano stark naked with a beanie on his head. The man never stopped playing once while I was trying to find out what was wrong with his cat. The nakedness didn't bother me as much as that beanie perched on his head, and the beanie didn't bother me as much as the fact that he couldn't stop with the piano long enough to discuss his cat. I turned and left.

I must have been in my musical phase, because less than a week later I ran into a somewhat similar incident, though in this case everyone had on clothes. I was calling on new clients again, this time in the West 8o's. They had a railroad apartment—one room right after the other like a string of railroad cars. No halls, no side rooms.

I found it odd that the door was open when I arrived and no one answered my ring. I entered and I immediately heard drums. Then I noticed the footprints painted on the ceiling and spotted signs labeling each room in pig Latin spelled backwards. I followed the sound of the drums and came upon the husband and wife sitting cross-legged on the floor, facing each other and beating bongo drums. They looked up when I entered the room, but they continued drumming. To give them credit, they did play more softly while we discussed their cat, but they never missed a beat.

They were still at it when I left the apartment. I never went back as I decided I couldn't compete with the drums.

There is a client of mine with two long-haired cats that she combs daily. Fine and good; nothing odd about that. In fact, I approve. But this lady saves every hair she combs out, and every hair the cats shed that she can get her hands on. Then she spins the cat hair into yarn and knits it into caps and scarves. With great pride, she gave me one of her cat hats. I suppose it was a great honor, but I had to give it away before I got home. It kicked off my allergies.

Barbara Baxley was preparing to go on tour with Tallulah Bankhead and Donald Cook in Noel Coward's *Private Lives* in 1949. It was no time to have a new cat, but a friend arrived with a gray-and-white kitten that had been found in a trashcan, and Barbara was hooked. This was the cat of hers I've mentioned in previous chapters.

Since the kitten was a female she named it Tula in honor of Miss Bankhead. If it had been a male, it would have been Donald for Mr. Cook.

Though the tour was to be a long one, almost a year on the road, Barbara had no intention of leaving Tula behind.

Luckily, Tula turned out to be an excellent train traveler. The problem was with hotels, most of which do not welcome pets. Short stays were fine because the hotel managers didn't catch on about the guest in Barbara's room. But on longer stops, it cost Barbara a small fortune in tips to maids and room service so they wouldn't snitch on Tula.

The big problem turned out to be Tula's litter-box needs. Barbara had always lived in circumstances that permitted her cats to be indoor-outdoor creatures, so a housebound—or hotel-bound—cat was a new experience to her. She didn't realize she could train the cat to use newspaper and she knew nothing about buying litter. So she did the next best thing. She began sneaking out into the halls of the hotels and taking sand from the ashtrays by the elevators.

At one hotel the management became quite concerned why sand was disappearing from the ashtrays near every elevator on every floor. An investigation began, and a maid, whom Barbara had tipped lavishly, cracked under pressure. Confronted by an irate hotel manager, Barbara confessed—and moved to another hotel.

I met Barbara and Tula when they returned from the tour of *Private Lives* when she called me to arrange to have her pet spayed. It was during Tula's recovery period that Barbara told me about the litter-box problems of traveling with a cat. Was there anything that could be done so that she could go on traveling with Tula?

I suggested we try to train her to use the tub. Tula turned out to be a brilliant student. First, we put her newspaper into the bathtub instead of a box. Tula got the message quickly and began to leap into the tub where the paper was when nature called.

When the paper was removed Tula continued to use the tub. Instead of worrying about litter and boxes, now all that was needed was a scooper to remove the feces for flushing down the toilet. A little scouring powder—nothing there to upset a hotel —and everything was right as rain again.

It was thanks to Barbara Baxley and Tula that I learned the trick of using booze as an antiseptic when giving injections. The time was 1953, when Barbara was appearing in Tennessee William's *Camino Real* at the National Theater on West 41st Street.

Tula had grown into a giant white-and-gray cat with a chronic bladder/kidney problem. It flared up late one morning of a matinee day. Barbara telephoned me to say that Tula was lying very still and felt very warm to the touch.

Because I couldn't get to Barbara's apartment before it was time for her to go to the theater, we agreed that she would take Tula with her and I would meet them backstage no later than 1 P.M., well ahead of Barbara's time to dress for the matinee performance.

When I got to the National—today it is the Trafalgar Theater —I told the stage doorman I had an appointment with Miss Baxley and we had to work fast. He glanced at my medical bag and took me straight to her dressing room.

I took one look at Tula and realized it was worse than Barbara had indicated over the telephone. Tula was lying on Barbara's dressing table as limp as an old fur boa. She didn't even move when she saw me, Camuti, the only enemy in the whole world from whom she usually ran as if shot from a cannon.

After a cursory examination, I turned to Barbara who had tears in her eyes. "I just don't know . . ."

Barbara cut me short. She pulled up her head, straightened her back and said with all the conviction of her training. "Don't say it. Give her the shots, do what you have to do. *She is going to be fine!*"

The shot was the first order of business. "Where can I get some boiling water to sterilize a syringe?" I asked Barbara.

She had nothing in her dressing room, so she sent me downstairs to the prop man's office. "I'm Dr. Camuti," I said. "Miss Baxley said you could get me some boiling water. I need it quickly."

He gave me a hot plate and an empty coffee can. Back in Barbara's dressing room, we boiled the hell out of the coffee can, tossed the water out, then boiled fresh water to sterilize the needle.

Then I realized we'd need alcohol for Tula's rump. Barbara had none. "Then how about some booze?"

Barbara felt terrible. She knew she should have kept some liquor in her dressing room for friends who came backstage after the show but she hadn't bothered. "Let me see what Jo Van Fleet has. She's a much better hostess than I."

Barbara went to the next dressing room and came back with a bottle of gin. Tula got her shot and pills.

That night, after the evening performance I met Barbara back at her apartment. Tula was showing signs of life again. "That's a pretty good cat," I said. "I think she'll be all right."

"All right?" said Barbara. "She'll be perfect."

Tula was never perfect, but she did recover from that particular bout. And I learned that liquor works very well in a pinch.

The finale to the story occurred backstage at the National when the prop man came up to Barbara Baxley, concerned for her health. He asked her how she was feeling.

"I'm fine," Barbara said.

"But the doctor . . . the injection."

"Oh, that was for my cat."

"A cat! You mean I stopped everything to get what he wanted for a cat?"

"Well, you don't think I'd have asked you to go to all that trouble for me, do you?"

Azadia Newman, a cousin of the Duchess of Windsor, is a fine portrait painter, much in demand on both sides of the Atlantic. It was a series of commissions in England that put her aboard the *Normandie* sailing from New York. Naturally Azadia took her green-eyed tabby, Dina, with her. It would not have occurred to her to go without Dina.

The trip went well and Dina enjoyed the delicacies brought to her several times a day by the cabin steward. But when the ship docked in England, the immigration official told her that Dina would have to stay in quarantine for six months. Azadia Newman hit the roof. She wouldn't hear of it. She never went anywhere without her cat, and she had no intention of staying in England for six months without Dina.

The immigration official said he was sorry, but rules were rules. Miss Newman said if that were the case, she would cancel all her portrait commissions, reboard the ship, and return to New York.

At that point, Captain Pugnet of the *Normandie* took Miss Newman aside. "Let Dina stay on board with me. She can share my cabin, I'll make certain she eats well, and I promise to take excellent care of her. Since I was not able to bring my own cat to sea, I assure you that you would be giving me great pleasure by leaving Dina with me." Dina herself sealed the deal in Miss Newman's mind by looking up at the captain and purring.

For the next six months Miss Newman worked at her portrait commissions and she kept a close watch on the *Normandie*'s arrivals in England. Each time the ship docked, Miss Newman shut up her studio and went to visit Dina.

While Dina expressed catlike pleasure at seeing her mistress again, there was no doubt in Miss Newman's mind that the tabby was thriving on her life at sea. She had the run of Captain Pugnet's quarters, was well fed, and somewhere along the way had acquired a handsome ribbon around her neck which she didn't seem to mind wearing.

When Miss Newman finished her work and reboarded the *Normandie* for her trip home, she saw that Dina had become something of a celebrity aboard ship. Every last deckhand knew her, and so did many of the passengers.

At a party midway across the Atlantic, José Iturbi, the famous pianist, played "Dinah" in her honor. Former Vice President John Nance Garner, also on board, invited Dina—and Miss Newman—to visit him at home. Dina loved every minute of it, and probably didn't miss seeing London at all.

Later, when Azadia Newman married Rouben Mamoulian, the Broadway and Hollywood director, I got to know him when they lived in New York City. Whether his wife turned him into a cat lover or he was one before they met I do not know. But he is certainly a cat lover today. In fact, he won't eat breakfast at their home in Beverly Hills without his cats sitting at the table. And he put a cat into every one of his movies, though sometimes you had to look hard to see it.

I once had a client, a Mrs. Elling, who owned a rather fancy art gallery. Her cat, Buster, on the other hand, was far from fancy, just an ordinary gray tabby. Or so I thought.

Actually, Buster was the cat's meow as I found out one evening when I finished treating him. Mrs. Elling suddenly said, "Would you like to see his dressing room?"

"His what?" I didn't believe I had heard what I heard.

"His dressing room. Come along."

Mrs. Elling led the way through the townhouse, which she and her husband had furnished in beautiful and expensive taste. On the third floor she ushered me into a room at the end of the hall that was more simply furnished than the rest. It was dominated by a large French armoire. She opened the top doors and started lifting tiny garments out of one of the drawers. "See?

Aren't they fine? They're all Buster's clothes, and this is where he dresses. This is his dressing room."

I considered the possibility that Mrs. Elling had a screw loose, but she was so matter-of-fact about it all that I didn't dare say a word. After all, if she wanted to dress her cat in tiny double-breasted suits, who was I to interfere?

"So this is where he dresses," I said, not knowing what else to say.

"He doesn't dress himself, you know. I help him. Or the maid does if I am out of the house."

I kept studying Mrs. Elling's face to see if she was kidding me. She wasn't. "But . . . er . . . he wasn't wearing anything when I saw him just now."

She looked at me as if I were a fool. "Of course not, why should he? He isn't going anywhere."

She proceeded to pull out all the cat-size garments: sports jackets, dinner clothes, three-piece suits. All of them were perfectly made with fine detailing from the buttonholes to the roll of the lapels.

"It's incredible," I said. "Those clothes look tailor made."

"Well of course they are." She gave me a scorching look. "How else could he get a decent fit?"

There were two warmhearted, totally cat-minded ladies in Mount Kisco who played a game with each other for years. It could have gone on for years longer if I had been the sort of doctor who was willing to collect double fees, which I would never do.

The ladies lived on opposite sides of Mount Kisco, and while I can't swear that they actually knew each other, they certainly knew about each other. One was Miss Tibbetts, a dietician at the Mount Kisco hospital. The other was Mrs. Gibson, a housewife. Each had her own house cats, and each kept cages in her backyard where she'd house neighborhood strays until she could find homes for them.

When one lady filled her cages she'd slip across town at night to the other lady's yard and leave the extra cat or two to be found the next morning. The recipient would then put the new strays into her cages until they filled up. Then *she* would make a night trip across town to deposit her extra cats.

Since they didn't speak to each other, neither Mrs. Gibson nor Miss Tibbetts knew that I had become the veterinarian for both of them. I caught on when Mrs. Gibson appeared in my office with a tiny golden tabby kitten for me to check. It was such a charmer that it stuck in my mind. I examined the kitten, who was perfectly fine except for ear mites, which I showed her how to treat. Mrs. Gibson begged me to think of someone who might give the kitten a home. I told her I'd try.

Unfortunately, kittens are easier to love than to find homes for, and I had no luck. I told Mrs. Gibson that when she called me about a week later.

"What am I going to do?" she said. "I just don't have room for another kitten."

I told her I'd keep trying, but I didn't offer much hope.

The next morning, Miss Tibbetts called me about finding a home for a beautiful golden tabby kitten she had found on her back steps. Her description rang a bell in my mind. I told her to bring the kitten to my office.

I recognized the kitten the moment I saw it. It was the one Mrs. Gibson had brought to me. Miss Tibbetts said, "Isn't it adorable, Dr. Camuti? Surely someone will want it. I suppose you ought to look it over while we're here just to make certain it's in good health."

"Don't worry, it is," I said.

Naturally, I had to explain how I knew. I thought Miss Tibbetts would be furious with Mrs. Gibson when I told her what that lady had been doing to her. Instead, Miss Tibbetts began to laugh. Then she confessed that she had been doing the same thing to Mrs. Gibson for years.

Now that the game had been exposed, it ended the late-night trips on the part of both ladies. I could have bitten my tongue off for ever exposing the cat caper, as I called it. Granted the

206

stray cats of Mount Kisco did a lot of late night traveling across town and back, but at each end of the trip there was a place to sleep, a good square meal, and a loving heart to care for them.

For wacky moments in the Camuti book of memories I think I'd have to give top honors to Mrs. Studebaker, whom I never met but will always remember.

I judged her to be a chatty lady from the long message she left with my answering service. The gist of it was that her cat was having urinary problems and she wanted to speak with the doctor.

From her voice, I got the impression of a sweet, elderly lady when I returned her call. She said that she was legally blind, though she did have partial vision—"Enough that I could see my cat—his name is Chilton—was having trouble with wee wee."

"Can you bring him to my office?" I said.

"That's not necessary any more, Doctor. I've cured him. I used to be a physical therapist. I'd be happy to tell you my technique, in case you want to use it."

"That's most kind of you," I said.

"Well, I remembered back to my early training. We had been taught that one way to reduce inflammation was to apply hot potato halves around the inflamed parts. Every time poor Chilton tried to wee wee I could see that his woosy-doosy was protruding but nothing came out. I decided it must be inflamed inside, which closed off the wee-wee tube. So I decided to use the hot-potato method on his woosy-doosy. Are you following me, Dr. Camuti?"

"Yes," I groaned, aching with sympathy pains for my fellow male creature. Not knowing what else to say I finally got up the gumption to ask, "What happened?"

"Oh," she said matter-of-factly in the same sweet little voice, "he flew through the air and pissed like hell!"

Chapter 18

PEOPLE ARE BORN and in time must die. Cats are born and in time they, too, must die. At my age I can look back on a great many deaths—of both people and cats—and all I can say is there is pain for those who go on living, and there is no way to measure the intensity of pain. Because man is higher up on the evolutionary scale than the cat doesn't necessarily mean that a man's death is more painful for those he leaves than for those who have lost a cat. Should one mourn more for an indifferent uncle than for a devoted and loving pet? I think it would be a strange person who did so.

Cat lovers will understand what I am saying. Non-pet people won't.

As a veterinarian it has often been my job to tell an owner it is time to let his pet die. Putting animals to sleep is routine work for any veterinarian, no matter what his specialty, but I can't say I go about it as comfortably as I do other phases of treatment. There is always that moment when you've got the syringe in your hand and you look down into the cat's eyes and know that you are about to make those eyes close for all time. It is never an easy moment for me. I have to remind myself that I am not playing God and deciding who shall live and who shall die, but a doctor who is 100 percent certain that nothing else can be done for his patient, that I am not just taking life but I am bringing a release from pain or from the miseries of old age to the cat. Only then can I go ahead.

Since death is a certainty, it always surprises me how many cat owners have never faced the moment and made plans. These are usually the same people who have never made any plans for what will happen when their own family members or they themselves die.

The facts are few and simple. When a cat is put to sleep by a veterinarian, he will dispose of the body unless the owner has plans for his cat's funeral himself. Should the cat die at home, then of course the disposal of the body is the owner's problem. Pet cemeteries are a good solution, and they exist all over the country. It's a wise owner who checks out the cemetery nearest his home while he can do it without the burden of grief.

People who live in the country, of course, have it a little easier than their city cousins. All that the country cat lover has to do is select a spot on his property and dig a hole. But make it a fairly deep hole so that no animal can come along and dig up your pet. I recommend a cardboard box, nothing very permanent, since I think along the Biblical lines of ashes to ashes.

City people can't arrange pet burials so easily. Open fields are not easily come by. But I've known several cat owners who were determined to give their pets proper send-offs and who carried out their plans.

One I learned about through a call from the FBI during World War II. The caller began by asking if I was indeed Dr. Louis J. Camuti, a veterinarian? I said I was. Did I know a Mr. Oskar Braun? I said I did.

Do you know him well? was the third question. "Not well," I said. "He's a local tradesman here in Mount Vernon. A nice guy, but he has a thick German accent that makes conversation a little difficult between us. I guess we've never gone beyond polite chitchat."

I thought that would end it, but the FBI man said, "What do you know about him?"

"Not much. He brought me a sick cat a few days ago, and

after I had examined it I told him that there was nothing that could be done so we agreed to put the cat to sleep. Mr. Braun asked to have the cat cremated and the ashes returned to him. I took care of that, and he picked up the ashes yesterday. I guess that's about it."

The agent thanked me, and asked that I come down to his office to identify Mr. Braun and the contents of the box he had been carrying at the time he had been brought in to the FBI.

I said I'd be right down. As I drove into Manhattan I kept trying to picture little Oskar Braun as someone dangerous enough to interest the FBI, but I couldn't do it. The thin balding man with the silver spectacles was just the man who sliced cold cuts in his delicatessen and sold packs of cigarettes. It was impossible to see him as anything else.

It turned out that I was right. I knew it the moment I saw the box he had been carrying at the "time of apprehension." It was the ashes containing all that was left of his beloved Gretchen. Mr. Braun told me the story he had already told the FBI agents several times. Only this time they accepted it.

Mr. Braun said that he always remembered how he had come to America by ship and the thrill he felt as he first looked up the Hudson River. It was a beautiful sight to him, and he wanted Gretchen's last moments on earth to be there. So he had taken a bus as close as he could get to the George Washington Bridge, and then continued on foot, carrying his little parcel of ashes. He decided that he would drop Gretchen's ashes from the exact center of the bridge so they would blow into the water instead of ending up on either shore.

Unfortunately, someone called the police and told them about a strange man with a little box on the bridge. They picked up Mr. Braun as he was saying his private farewell to Gretchen before opening the box.

Between his anguish over Gretchen and his confusion and fright at being arrested, his accent became impossible for the police to decipher. They turned him over to the FBI, who thought he might be a German spy about to blow up the bridge or drop poison into the Hudson River.

By the time I arrived, Mr. Braun had calmed down enough for the FBI to understand his story. But they still had to have that stuff in the box identified. I couldn't help wondering what Gretchen would have thought about the trouble her ashes had caused. I imagine she'd have laughed her cat head off at finding herself, a gentle lady in life, a risk to national security in death.

I always thought of Mrs. Callaghan as a kind, soft-spoken lady, somewhere in her eighties. But when I received an invitation to attend the wake for her cat, Molly, who had died of old age, I learned there was a lot more to Mrs. Callaghan than met the eye. There was still a feisty woman inside that frail body and a mind capable of some very fancy scheming.

Since I had always liked Mrs. Callaghan and Molly, I felt honored to be invited to Molly's wake, which was attended by Mrs. Callaghan's own doctor and nurse, the head of the local humane society, and a few friends. Molly's body rested in a small white casket in the center of the room. Tea and sherry were served, nothing stronger. "This is very nice," I said to Mrs. Callaghan, "and what are you going to do with the body?"

"I'm going to have Molly buried with me."

"Well, before you get your heart set on it," I told her, "you'd better check with the cemetery authorities to see if it's okay."

Mrs. Callaghan called me the next day to say that she had called the cemetery in Pennsylvania where her family plot was located and they told her it wouldn't be allowed. Instead—or at the time I thought it was an alternate plan—Mrs. Callaghan arranged for cremation in New York City. She asked me, as Molly's doctor, if I could pick up the casket and take it to the crematory as she couldn't do it. I said I would.

That Sunday, I brought Molly's ashes to Mrs. Callaghan. "Now, what are you going to do with her ashes?" I asked.

Mrs. Callaghan smiled. "I told you that Molly was going to be buried with me."

I wondered if Mrs. Callaghan's mind wasn't slipping a bit. "But you told me your cemetery wouldn't permit it."

Another smile. "I've arranged to be buried in my wedding

dress. They can't stop that. And I'm going to have Molly's ashes sewn into the hem of my gown."

Which is exactly what happened.

Offhand I'd guess there are many pets buried in people cemeteries. When their dog, Bootsie, died of an internal hemorrhage, Mr. and Mrs. Lewis had him cremated and then discovered it was too painful living with his ashes. Knowing that the cemetery where their family plot was located would not accept Bootsie's ashes, they solved the problem very simply. They took the ashes to the cemetery and pretended to be visiting a relative's grave. While Mrs. Lewis kept watch, Mr. Lewis dug a hole under the cement bench that had been placed at their plot and interred Bootsie's ashes there. They both find it comforting to know that Bootsie is waiting for them.

Charles and Janice Remsen, who live on a houseboat in Florida, wrote to tell me how they have handled the situation. Their solution is a complete reversal of the one arrived at by Mrs. Callaghan and the Lewises. When the Remsens learned that their cat, Kali, could not be buried in a human cemetery, they arranged with the American Pet Memorial Cemetery in Fort Lauderdale to take Kali's ashes. But the thought of Kali being alone bothered them, so they called Kenneth S. Waite, the proprietor of Kali's cemetery and asked if when the time comes their own ashes could be buried near Kali's. Mr. Waite told them it was perfectly legal, and arrangements have been made.

I doubt if there has been a cat owner since the dawn of time who has not attributed emotions to his or her cat. The emotions, of course, are always human emotions, but are they really there at all? When a cat dies, the humans who loved it suffer, but does another cat? The truth is that even a cat who has shared its home with another cat may not miss that cat at all when it dies. After all, cats are loners.

Yet, having said all this, I still think of Green-eyes and Marigold and their behavior at cat funerals. I can only tell the stories. I can't really explain them.

When their gray cat, Monkey, became incurably ill and it was agreed that I would put him to sleep, Maurice Dolbier asked that I have the body cremated and the ashes returned. I followed instructions and sent Monkey's body to a crematory after he was put to sleep. I returned the ashes to the Dolbiers, whose daughter had carefully thought out funeral plans. Monkey's ashes would be taken to Mr. Dolbier's mother's house in Maine and buried in the backyard.

Maurice Dolbier told me what happened in Maine. On the day of the funeral the family gathered on the back porch with Monkey's ashes. They were trying to decide which spot in the backyard would be Monkey's final resting place when Green-eyes, Grandmother Dolbier's stately female cat, pushed her way out through the screen door. With just a quick glance over her shoulder to signal the family to follow her, Green-eyes left the porch and led the family to a spot way in the back of the yard. She stopped in front of the place she had chosen. She sat down and waited while Maurice Dolbier dug the hole and placed Monkey's ashes in it. When he had covered the hole, he turned to Green-eyes, who had watched the whole procedure in silence. "Would you care to say a few words?"

It was his attempt to lighten the atmosphere, nothing more, but to everyone's amazement Green-eyes did speak. Then, without further ado, she stood up and turned to the house. She glanced back again to make certain her meaning was understood and then she led the mourners back to the house.

Pansy and Marigold were mother and daughter calicos who lived with Dean and Beverley Fuller and their two children, John and Liza. The calicos commuted every weekend from the Fuller apartment in Manhattan to their country house in Connecticut. In the city they were contented apartment cats, but once they reached the house in Connecticut they took off for outdoor adventures.

One Saturday afternoon, Marigold came home, but Pansy didn't. It bothered the Fullers, since Pansy usually kept fairly regular hours. They grew more and more worried as the sun began to set. All four Fullers went to different parts of their large property calling for Pansy, but there wasn't a sign of her.

All through the night Dean and Beverly listened for the familiar tap-tap on their bedroom window that would mean Pansy had come home and wanted to be let in. It was a system of Pansy's own devising that she had worked out on those rare occasions when she had stayed out for a late-night romp. Her system was to climb the grape arbor, leap from it to the roof, then walk around to the window of the master bedroom and tap and scratch on it until someone opened it for her.

But on this night Pansy never came home.

In the morning, the Fuller children found her body on the road not far from the house. Pansy had died in running position. It looked as if she had taken a nap in the middle of the little-traveled road, suddenly been awakened by an oncoming car, and killed before she could leap out of the way.

The Fullers chose a remote and quite corner of their garden for Pansy, and they buried her there.

Several hours later, as Beverley was going out to her herb garden, Marigold decided to go out, too. She gave an odd meow that made Beverley turn to look at her. There was something in that meow that somehow told Beverley that Marigold wanted her to follow.

Though she hadn't attended her mother's funeral, Marigold led Beverley straight to her mother's grave, where she sat down, looked up at Beverley and began to purr. Beverley felt that Marigold was trying to comfort her by telling her that she was still with her. Beverley burst into tears and ran to the house.

It was the only time, to any of the Fullers' knowledge, that Marigold ever visited her mother's grave or made reference to it.

Loving your cat is one thing but going overboard is something else, and the lady I am thinking about went about as far overboard as anyone can.

It began with a call from the woman in Westchester saying she wanted me to come see her cat. Having attended to that cat before and never having had the impression that there was anything wacky about the client, I went. I didn't even ask what was wrong over the telephone.

When I got to her apartment in White Plains I was floored to see a baby-sized white casket set up in the center of the living room. The cat was in it, dead, and there were flowers all around.

"What's this?" I asked the woman.

"Well, you were his doctor, and I thought you'd want to see him after he died." She said it very matter-of-factly.

So I paid my respects and I made them brief, as I couldn't wait to get out of there. The woman offered to pay me for my visit, but I refused.

The woman accompanied me to the door. She was with me as we passed through a darkened room I hadn't paid any attention to on the way in. I think it was because my eyes were fixed on that white casket up ahead. But this time, I realized it was a bedroom. A thin sliver of afternoon sun came through the closed curtains and I could see there was someone in the bed.

I couldn't really see the person, but there was something very white and still about the person. "Who's that?" I asked.

Again that matter-of-fact voice. "It's my mother. She died and I haven't had time to bury her."

I couldn't believe my ears. The woman had had time to get a casket and flowers for her cat, but she hadn't had time to take care of her mother! If I hadn't gotten out of that apartment quickly, I think I'd have wrapped my medical bag around that woman's head.

Tailless Tom has been gone a long time now, but I still see him in my mind's eye as clear as if he had only died yesterday. I see him strutting along proud as punch, his rear end with only the tiniest stump of tail on it twitching in the breeze, and I can still smile and choke up. I like to think of Tailless Tom as my cat, which he was, but he wasn't—the way the Statue of Liberty

215

belongs to me, but it doesn't. The truth is that Tailless Tom belonged to a whole regiment, and I think every man in that regiment belonged to him.

Tailless Tom's proud way of walking might make you think he was a Manx cat, but he wasn't. He was just an ordinary brown alley cat who had lost his tail—he never told me how—in his early years before we met. That was back in the early 1930's when I first opened my hospital in Mount Vernon.

Tom lived near the hospital with a nice but terribly squeamish lady who couldn't stand the things Tom brought home from his daily outings in the fields that used to be plentiful around Mount Vernon.

Because he was such a friendly, gregarious cat who seemed to truly like people, Tom dropped in on me one day and I showed him around my hospital, which stood clean and empty while I waited for customers to discover me. After the tour, Tom was kind enough to accept a dish of baby beef before going on his way.

Shortly afterward, I met the lady he lived with. She dropped in for some advice about Tom. Was there any way she could stop him from bringing home the mice, moles and birds he caught? "He puts them right at my feet, Dr. Camuti, and sometimes they're still alive!"

I told her she should feel complimented. And she should be proud that her cat was such a good hunter.

She sniffed at that, and dabbed at her eyes with a lacy handkerchief. "Well, I can't stand it. I'm a very nervous woman and I find it upsetting."

The woman knew that I thought Tailless Tom was a terrific cat. That was why she called me a week later. She sounded close to hysteria. "Do you want Tom? He's yours right now. I can't take it anymore."

"What happened?"

Her voice rose, and the words came tumbling out in a wild rush. "Do you know where he is this very minute? Sitting outside the screened porch door with a snake in his mouth, and it's still alive! You have to come and get him right away, Dr. Camuti, or I'll find some other way to get rid of him. I can't have this happening anymore!"

I said I'd be right over. Sure enough, there was Tom sitting exactly where she said he was. The snake turned out to be a racer, absolutely harmless and a baby, not much larger than a big worm. Tom dropped it at my feet. I patted his head, and the snake shot off into the grass.

I brought Tom back with me to the hospital. He immediately sensed it was his new home, and he never went back to visit his former home. I told Tom that the hospital would have to be a temporary home for him, because as my practice grew the hospital was bound to fill up with all sorts of animals, and a cat in residence just wouldn't work out. I told him that I would certainly do my darnedest to find him a good, permanent home. Tom said nothing. He just rubbed against my pants leg and purred.

With his personality, I thought I'd have no trouble in finding a home for Tailless Tom. People seemed interested when I told them about the cat's warm, friendly disposition, but when I got to the part about his talents as a hunter I lost many of them. And the one or two that asked to meet Tom didn't seem to find this tailless wonder as attractive as I did.

One day, I thought of a perfect solution. I was the commanding officer at the White Plains Armory on South Broadway. There were lots of people around over there, and Tom liked people. It would be a great home for him. There were plenty of open fields around the place so Tom would have good hunting.

Tom took to army life like a duck to water, and the men fell for him. One of the sergeants made him his own dog tag and put it on a chain around his neck. Wearing the proof of how special he was, Tom strutted more proudly than ever.

Tom's favorite time was when the 102nd Medical Regiment would move out to Camp Smith, near Peekskill, New York, for two weeks each summer. As a member of the regiment, Tom naturally went along.

As commanding officer of the Service Command at Camp Smith, one of my duties was to supply the food to the thirteen companies in the regiment. All the supply sergeants tried to give special treats to Tom as a way of pleasing me, but Tom let them know he couldn't be bought. He would just turn up his nose and march on.

Though he wasn't officially assigned to the job, Tom made mess hall inspection his job. It was a big job, since there were eleven mess halls for the enlisted men and two for the officers, all strung out in a 400-foot line. Tom would drop by many of them two or three times a day to look things over. Obviously he had his favorite kitchens, and the men who ran them felt honored by Tom's visits. Those he ignored tried desperately to lure him over, as though Tailless Tom was in charge of bestowing some terrific award, like the Duncan Hines Seal of Approval.

Tom actually made the whole camp his command, but he would always check in at my company several times a day just to give me a rub and a purr and let me know that I still stood high in his affection. But he refused to sleep in my officer's tent.

Tom was a born diplomat. He always bedded down with the enlisted men.

When we returned from Camp Smith, Tom went back to hunting the open fields around the armory. No matter how far he wandered, he always kept the armory in his sights, and the minute he saw men gathering for a meeting, he came racing back.

Life went on for Tom at the armory for several years. And then one day, coming back from one of his field patrols, he was run over by a car right in front of the armory. It was a loss that every man felt.

There was no question about Tom's funeral. It was automatically decided that he should have a full military send-off.

I don't think there was one man attached to the armory who skipped Tom's funeral. He was placed in a small casket and buried in the front yard of the armory while a military salute was fired in his honor and taps was sounded. I looked down the line of men standing at attention as Tailless Tom went to his glory, and I could see the sun picking up wet spots on many faces. I admit the tears were running freely down my face.

Today there is a small marker on Tailless Tom's grave in the front yard of the armory. I often stop when I'm driving to pause a minute and look at Tom's grave and remember him. I can still hear the sound of his dog tag rubbing against the chain around his neck as he strutted around with his stump of tail high in the air, and all four feet marching in proud cadence. He was a great cat and a good soldier.

EPILOGUE

At this point I picture the reader smacking his or her lips waiting for old Camuti to tell his greatest cat story. I'm sorry but I don't have one. Or maybe I've already told it. It's even possible that I've forgetten the best cat story I ever had.

The truth is that I don't think I have one best cat story, at least not in the way a dog lover could come up with one. No cat ever went up into the Alps with a keg of brandy around its neck to rescue anybody. Cats don't leap into raging streams to rescue devoted masters, and they don't rush into fiery buildings to save children.

It's not that cats care less about the people who love them; they just care differently. You can ask for love from a dog and you'll get it. Wise cat owners know to give love, and to recognize its return in little ways. Or put it this way: With dogs and people it's love in big splashy colors. When you're involved with a cat you're dealing in pastels. I like that about cats.

I like the fact that when a cat decides to lick my hand I know that cat truly likes me. With a dog, who can tell? Maybe the dog has been taught to lick an outstretched hand, maybe it wants to be petted, or maybe the dog smells the roast beef sandwich I had for lunch. With a cat there is never any doubt. I am liked —maybe not loved, but liked—at least for the moment.

Granted, among the thousands of cats who have been my patients, there have been very few hand-lickers. In fact, there have been very few who stuck around when I made my appearance. But I like that about cats. Would you stick around if you thought the man coming through the door was going to hurt you? I wouldn't, and I can't blame a cat for not wanting to, either.

I think a lot of what I like about cats has to do with the way I was brought up. In my day, you shook hands when you met someone, and when you left you said goodbye politely. Kissing was only for very special people. Nowadays, it's all kissing—and not only with the show-business people who have been my clients. People kiss hello and they kiss goodbye, and it can be with people they hardly know. Well, I still like a little formality. When I kiss somebody it is because they mean something to me, and I hope that when and if they kiss me it is because I mean something to them.

It's that appreciation of formality that makes me like cats. They are perfectly willing to keep their distance with strangers until they decide about them, and they'd just as soon that people would respond in kind.

I like dogs, dachshunds especially. But I trust and respect cats more. I think everything that I like and admire about cats is what has caused them so much trouble through the centuries. It is their impenetrable dignity, the great silence you can feel about them, their way of looking at a person without ever revealing what they are thinking that has unnerved mankind and led to all sorts of ridiculous connections between cats, the devil and witchcraft.

But cats have survived it all, from ancient Egypt to the present day, and I have no doubt that they will go on surviving. It is my opinion that the people who hate cats, fear them or don't trust them are people who are unsure of themselves. Deep down inside, where they may never have to face it, they are jealous when they see a cat going about its business, indifferent to what anyone wants or expects of it. That cat is leading its own life, giving affection only to whom it wants, accepting affection only when and from whom it chooses. If I were someone who spent his life putting up with and giving in to people I had doubts about, I think I might want to kick the stuffings out of a cat that was showing me it could lead a life I didn't have the guts to.

Sure, I've met a lot of wacky cat owners, some weak and some strong, but I suspect that underneath it all they must be self-sufficient people. Their cat says that to me. If those people needed a pet that would give them wild displays of affection every time they came in the door, they'd have picked a different pet. Cats are for people who have some self-contentment.

So I haven't got one last great cat story. But maybe, if you see things the way I do, every cat is a great story within itself. I only know that I can look back with fondness on a life spent tending to cats. Though they didn't give me much affection in return for my work, I have no doubt that they knew I was trying to help them. Cats are too bright not to know. And if it is not their way to show a little appreciation, I can understand that. I've been told so often that I'm a pretty crusty old bird that I accept it as truth.

There have been many a time when I've choked up at an unexpected kindness and said nothing. Later on, I wanted to kick myself. Well, maybe there are cats walking around today wanting to kick themselves for hissing and spitting at Camuti when he was only trying to help them. I hope so.

Not that it really matters, because as long as the good Lord lets us, Alex and I will be heading out late in the afternoon making our way to our patients. Who knows? One of the Oswillas or Nicodemuses I have yet to meet may be that great cat story I would like to have told here.

But I don't really expect that to happen. It will be more than enough for me if one day I open a door and find a cat sitting in the middle of the room looking up and waiting for me.

Come to think of it, that would be a great cat story.